ARTHRITIS

Diagnosis & Treatments

2016 Report

A Special Report
published by the editors of
Arthritis Advisor
in conjunction with
Cleveland Clinic

Arthritis: Diagnosis & Treatments

Consulting Editor: Steven Maschke, MD, Department of Orthopaedic Surgery, Orthopaedic and Rheumatologic Institute, Cleveland Clinic;
Linda Mileti, MD, Department of Rheumatologic and Immunologic Disease, Cleveland Clinic

Author: Doug Mazanec
Group Directors, Belvoir Media Group: Diane Muhlfeld, Jay Roland
Creative Director, Belvoir Media Group: Judi Crouse
Belvoir Editor: Kate Brophy
Contributing Editor: Jim Black
Illustrations: Alayna Paquette, Thinkstock, Dreamstime, Creative Commons

Publisher, Belvoir Media Group: Timothy H. Cole

ISBN: 978-1-879620-76-6

To order additional copies of this report or for customer service questions, please call 877-300-0253, go to www.arthritis-advisor.com/products, or write Health Special Reports, 535 Connecticut Avenue, Norwalk, CT 06854-1713.

NEW FINDINGS

- Weight may influence odds of RA remission (Page 10, Box 1-4)

- Treat-to-target approach may lower RA mortality risk (Page 14, Box 1-7)

- Hand OA linked to cardiac risks (Page 20, Box 2-3)

- Drugs may reduce cardiovascular risks in RA patients (Page 20, Box 2-4)

- Women with RA more likely to die from respiratory and other causes (Page 21, Box 2-5)

- Acetaminophen ineffective for back pain (Page 26, Box 3-1)

- Steroid injections may hurt your hips (Page 30, Box 3-4)

- Opioids linked to abnormal heart rhythm (Page 31, Box 3-5)

- Methotrexate/biologic combo helps save large joints (Page 36, Box 3-6)

- Tapering, stopping RA treatment may be feasible (Page 41, Box 3-7)

- Injections helpful for knee OA (Page 42, Box 3-8)

- Arthroscopic surgery no help for mild knee OA (Page 49, Box 4-3)

- "Prehab" may reduce need for postoperative care after joint replacement (Page 53, Box 4-6)

- Two-week return to driving for most hip-replacement patients (Page 59, Box 4-8)

- Long-term results favorable for lumbar disc replacement (Page 65, Box 4-13)

- Studies support benefits of glucosamine and chondroitin (Page 71, Box 5-1)

- Higher vitamin D levels linked to lower OA pain (Page 75, Box 5-3)

- Real acupuncture no better than fake treatment for knee pain (Page 76, Box 5-4)

- Acupuncture provides short-term help for chronic back pain (Page 77, Box 5-5)

- Spinal manipulation may ease back-related leg pain (Page 78, Box 5-7)

- Wine may help your knees, but beer may be harmful (Page 82, Box 5-8)

- Exercise, manual therapy help with OA (Page 87, Box 6-2)

- Running may protect against knee OA (Page 90, Box 6-4)

- Sustained weight loss relieves knee OA pain (Page 92, Box 6-6)

- Knee brace may ease OA pain (Page 95, Box 6-8)

INTRODUCTION

If you're among the one in five American adults with arthritis, you have a constant and unwanted companion. Arthritis encompasses more than 100 diseases that can limit your activity during the day and keep you up at night, eating away at your joints and eroding your quality of life.

Given that arthritis is anticipated to affect a quarter of the U.S. population by 2030 and no cure has been found, it's not surprising that countless research hours and millions of dollars are being spent on ways to manage this joint-robbing disease. Researchers are exploring new non-surgical treatments for osteoarthritis (OA, the most common form of arthritis), while continuing their quest for a disease-modifying drug to arrest OA progression. They're improving joint replacements and other surgeries that can alleviate OA pain and restore function, and fine-tuning diagnostic methods and treatment strategies that place more people with rheumatoid arthritis (RA) on the path to remission while minimizing their risk of complications.

This report summarizes some of the latest research into the two main types of arthritis, OA and RA. Here's a guide to what's inside:

- Chapter 1: We examine the development of OA and RA, the risk factors for these diseases, and the goals of treatment.
- Chapter 2: A look at the clinical, laboratory, and imaging tests used to diagnose arthritis, as well as potential complications of OA and RA that may occur beyond the joints.
- Chapter 3: An overview of the broad array of medications and drug combinations used to treat arthritis, from oral medicines and topical treatments to potent infusions and injections.
- Chapter 4: A guide to joint surgery, including the risks and benefits of joint replacements and advice on when to consider surgery.
- Chapter 5: We enter the world of complementary and alternative medicine, to review which supplements, mind/body therapies, and other less traditional treatments may help with arthritis.
- Chapter 6: What can you do to avoid arthritis or minimize its effects on your life? We examine preventive and coping strategies.

Keep in mind that some of the treatments discussed may still be investigational and not yet available. New therapies sometimes require many years to be proven safe and effective before they're available at your doctor's office.

We hope this report, now in its 13th edition, will guide you in managing your arthritis care, so that you can make arthritis a companion you can tolerate, or even abandon.

ABOUT CLEVELAND CLINIC

Cleveland Clinic, located in Cleveland, Ohio, is a nonprofit, multispecialty academic medical center that integrates clinical and hospital care with research and education. Founded in 1921, Cleveland Clinic is one of the largest and most respected hospitals in the country today, recognized as one of the best hospitals in America by *U.S. News & World Report* every year since the magazine began rating hospitals in 1990. Cleveland Clinic's orthopaedic and rheumatologic programs consistently rank among the top three in the country.

Cleveland Clinic's Orthopaedic & Rheumatologic Institute brings together all healthcare providers who treat musculoskeletal impairments, including arthritis, osteoporosis, metabolic bone diseases, immunologic diseases of the connective tissues, athletic injuries, bone fractures, musculoskeletal cancer, and congenital and pediatric diseases.

More than 100 physicians, orthopaedic surgeons, and physical therapists manage more than 250,000 patient visits, and perform more than 14,000 surgical procedures annually. Using innovative joint replacement and reconstructive methods, Cleveland Clinic's orthopaedic surgeons reconstruct thousands of hand, wrist, elbow, shoulder, foot, ankle, hip, and knee joints each year.

Cleveland Clinic's Department of Rheumatic and Immunologic Diseases has a long history of excellence and innovation in the care of patients with illnesses such as osteoporosis, osteoarthritis, rheumatoid arthritis, fibromyalgia, bursitis, vasculitis, lupus, and chronic fatigue syndrome.

TABLE OF CONTENTS

TABLE OF CONTENTS

ARTHRITIS: A BROAD RANGE OF DISEASES

About 60 percent of adults over age 60 have joint degeneration as revealed by X-rays.

What is a joint?

In more than 130 places around your body, two or more bones come together to form a joint. Covering the ends of these bones is cartilage, a smooth, slippery tissue that lets the bones move easily and comfortably against one another (see Box 1-1, "Anatomy of a knee joint").

Each joint is enclosed in a capsule made of sturdy connective tissue. The capsule has a thin lining, the synovium, which secretes fluid to nourish and lubricate the cartilage and maintain its health.

Muscles, tendons, and ligaments surrounding the joint help maintain the alignment between bones, keeping the joint stable, holding it together, and making sure that any forces or stress that occur during movement take place across parts such as the cartilage, which is best suited to handle and cushion such forces. Cartilage acts as a kind of shock absorber for your joints by changing shape when compressed, then regaining its normal shape when the load is gone. By lubricating the joint surfaces and absorbing force, cartilage protects underlying bone, which would otherwise wear away from friction.

What is osteoarthritis?

Over time, cartilage loses much of its elasticity and strength and becomes more likely to tear and split when stressed. As a result, its cushioning properties diminish, leading to the most common form of arthritis: osteoarthritis (OA), or "wear and tear" arthritis (see Box 1-2, "Stages of osteoarthritis in the knee"). About 60 percent of adults over age 60 have joint degeneration as revealed by X-rays. Though it most often occurs in weight-bearing joints such as the hips, knees, ankles, and spine, OA can affect the shoulders, hands, and feet.

What are the risk factors for OA?

A combination of factors makes a person more likely to develop osteoarthritis:

BOX 1-1

ANATOMY OF A KNEE JOINT

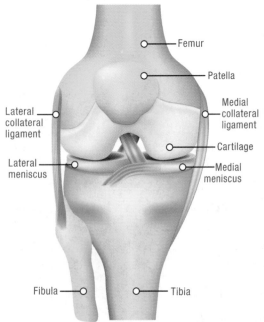

- Femur
- Patella
- Medial collateral ligament
- Lateral collateral ligament
- Cartilage
- Lateral meniscus
- Medial meniscus
- Fibula
- Tibia

- **Obesity:** The more you weigh, the more stress you put on your ankles, hips, knees, and spine. It's estimated that each additional pound of body weight puts three extra pounds of stress on your knees as you walk. Losing weight lowers your risk for OA, and may help slow the development of the disease once you get it. Research indicates that excess weight contributes to the risks of knee injury and future OA.

- **Injury:** Previous injury to a joint seems to put you at higher risk of developing post-traumatic arthritis in that joint later on.

- **Overuse:** If your daily behavior involves repeated, heavy use of a joint, especially accompanied by bending, then you are at higher risk of developing arthritis in that joint. This is especially true of the spine and the knee.

- **Genetics:** Some people are born with defects in the cells (chondrocytes) needed to make and maintain the collagen that is a key component of joint cartilage. Research published in 2015 in *Osteoarthritis and Cartilage* found that among 220 people, ages 26 to 61, those with one or more parents who underwent total knee replacement for severe OA were more likely to experience worsening knee pain and cartilage loss over 10 years.

- **Anatomy:** Some studies suggest that certain abnormalities in your anatomy—including unequal leg lengths and flat feet—may lead to problems with OA.

- **Smoking:** Smoking has been linked to greater cartilage loss and more pain in people who already have OA.

- **Diabetes:** People with type 2 diabetes are at greater risk of OA, although obesity (a prime type 2 diabetes risk factor) may be more to blame than the diabetes itself. Still, a study published in the February 2015 issue of *Arthritis Care & Research* found that among 530 people (average age 65) with hand OA, those with type 2 diabetes had more severe hand pain and tenderness.

What is rheumatoid arthritis?

Rheumatoid arthritis (RA) is an autoimmune disease of the joint lining, or synovium, and is the most common form of inflammatory arthritis.

In RA, a faulty immune system engages in "friendly fire," triggering a gradual destructive attack on the joints, as well as on organs throughout the body. The joint lining becomes inflamed

BOX 1-2

STAGES OF OSTEOARTHRITIS IN THE KNEE

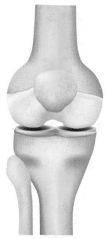

Healthy knee
Intact cartilage provides a smooth sliding surface to protect the ends of bones.

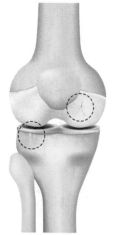

Beginning stage
Cartilage begins to wear down.

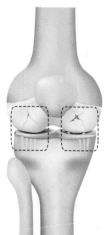

Moderate knee OA
Considerable loss of cartilage and moderate inflammation.

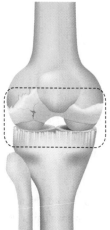

Advanced stage
Total loss of cartilage, bone spurs, severe inflammation.

BOX 1-3

HEALTHY KNEE VS. KNEE WITH RA

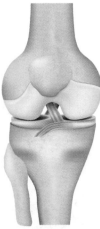 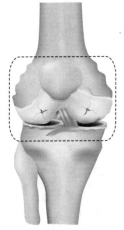

Healthy knee
No swelling in joint lining. Cartilage is intact, protecting the ends of the bones and allowing them to roll, rotate, and glide smoothly against and over each other.

RA knee
Inflammation and swelling of the joint lining. Cartilage is eaten away by enzymes in the joint. Bone erodes.

NEW FINDING

BOX 1-4

Weight may influence odds of RA remission

People with rheumatoid arthritis (RA) who are overweight or underweight are significantly less likely than their normal-weight peers to achieve remission, a recent study suggests. Among the 944 RA patients who were followed for three years, those who were morbidly obese—body mass index (BMI) of 35 or higher—were 50 to 64 percent less likely than those of normal weight (BMI 18.5 to 24.9) to achieve sustained RA remission. Also, the odds of achieving remission were 25 percent and 45 percent lower, respectively, among overweight (BMI 25 to 29.9) and underweight study participants (BMI less than 18.5), the study found.

American College of Rheumatology Annual Meeting, November 2014

and swollen, releasing enzymes into the joint capsule that, over time, eat away at the bone and cartilage. As the cartilage is destroyed, the cushion between bones is lost, and the bone rubbing against bone becomes increasingly painful (see Box 1-3, "Healthy knee vs. knee with RA").

Damage to joints occurs relatively rapidly in RA. Some research indicates that 90 percent of patients show bone erosion in the hand or foot joints within the first few years of developing the disease.

What are the risk factors for rheumatoid arthritis?

Though the precise causes of RA are unclear, several factors may increase your risk:

▶ Being female: Though it can affect anyone, including children, RA affects women twice as often as men. What's more, research suggests that women with early RA may be less likely than men to achieve sustained remission.

▶ Getting older: The incidence of RA increases with age, with onset usually occurring between 30 and 50 years of age.

▶ Infection: There is some suggestion that exposure to an infection, such as a virus or bacterium, may cause an abnormal immune system reaction in those who are already susceptible to RA, thus triggering the disease. One study found that people with new-onset RA had greater numbers of an intestinal bacterium, Prevotella copri, compared to healthy people or patients with chronic, treated RA. Other studies have suggested a link between Porphyromonas gingivalis, the main infectious agent associated with periodontal disease, and the development of RA.

▶ Obesity: Emerging evidence has identified a potential link between obesity and the development of RA. Studies also suggest that obese patients are less likely to achieve early control of their RA, and that weight may play a role in determining whether RA will go into remission (see Box 1-4, "Weight may influence odds of RA remission"). Like RA, obesity has been linked to inflammation, and fat tissues and cells produce substances involved in inflammation and immunity.

▶ Genetics: Inheriting specific genes may make you more likely to develop RA. For instance, HLA-DR4, a genetic marker associated with RA, is found in as many as 60 to 70 percent of Caucasians with the disease, compared to only 30 percent of the general population. And in a study published April 28, 2015, in the *Journal of the American Medical Association*, researchers reported that variations on the HLA-DRB1 gene could predict disease severity, response to treatment, and risk of death in RA patients.

‣ **Inflammatory pathways:** Proteins known as cytokines are involved in inflammatory diseases such as RA. Some are inflammatory, while others have anti-inflammatory properties. Some research has identified an imbalance of pro-inflammatory and anti-inflammatory cytokines in RA patients.

‣ **Smoking:** Use of tobacco has been directly linked with an increased risk for developing RA, and with greater disease severity. A 2014 study found that RA patients who smoked were more than twice as likely as their non-smoking counterparts to experience a rapid progression of their disease within the first year of diagnosis. Adding salt to the mix may make things worse: A 2014 study found an association between high sodium intake and greater RA risk among smokers, but not non-smokers. On a positive note, some evidence suggests that compared to those who continue to smoke, RA patients who quit smoking may see improvements in joint tenderness, swelling, stiffness, and disease activity.

‣ **Gum disease:** Emerging research continues to uncover an association between gum (periodontal) disease and RA. Both conditions are characterized by damage from a wayward immune response and inflammation.

OA and RA: Common symptoms

No matter which form of arthritis you have, the disease can cause pain, swelling, stiffness, loss of motion, and deformity (such as bone loss or bone spurs). Once the arthritis becomes advanced, it can erode the joint cartilage enough to let bone rub against bone. This rubbing is usually painful because, unlike cartilage, bone contains nerves.

‣ **Pain in the joint:** Localized pain is the chief symptom of both OA and RA. In the early stages, the pain might be occasional, yet worsens with activity. The pain level often can vary, with days or weeks of no pain followed by periods of continual

BOX 1-5

In addition to the common symptoms listed on the previous page and at right, people with RA can have the following symptoms:

- Symmetrical pain: RA usually begins in the joints of your hands and feet, and often affects the same joint on both sides of the body.

- Episodic flare-ups: RA is characterized by episodic flare-ups, which result in severely swollen, red, hot, and tender joints. The disease may lie dormant for a number of years and then return.

- Effects on the entire body: People with RA often have body-wide, or systemic, symptoms such as fatigue, general discomfort, and loss of appetite.

- Prolonged morning stiffness: People with RA often feel very stiff in the morning for several hours. Stiffness is also present in OA, but does not typically last as long.

discomfort. Often the pain gets worse when you are exposed to reduced barometric pressure, such as the kind that may happen if the weather is bad, and which occurs during an extended airplane flight.

- **Loss of mobility:** As arthritis advances, the mobility in the affected joint diminishes.

- **Noisy joints:** As cartilage is lost from the ends of your bones, the movement of bone against bone, or sliding of ligaments along bone, is no longer smooth, but can cause clicking, grinding, or popping noises.

- **Swelling around the joint:** The irritation of bone rubbing against bone, or the inflammation of the joint lining and surrounding tissue due to a faulty immune response, can cause the joint to swell and become red and tender to the touch.

- **Reduced strength:** Because people with painful arthritis often limit their activity, the muscles, ligaments, and tendons around a joint don't get sufficient exercise, and muscle strength decreases.

See also Box 1-5, "RA symptoms," and Box 1-6, "OA symptoms."

OA: Treatment goals and strategies

The goals of treating osteoarthritis (OA) are to reduce pain and stiffness, improve mobility in the affected joint, stabilize the joint, slow down the gradual destruction of cartilage and bone, and restore your ability to get on with your day-to-day life.

OA is typically treated with a combination of approaches, including:

- Exercise and stretching
- Application of heat and cold to the joint
- Physical therapy
- Rest
- Weight control
- Support devices, such as braces, canes, or crutches
- Medications (oral, topical, and injectable)
- Surgery, to bring relief if all else fails

Newer methods of treating OA include finding ways to slow or halt the breakdown of cartilage. The search for such disease-modifying OA drugs continues, and although some drugs have shown some potential, at this point there is no proven way to halt or reverse the disease process once it has started.

The American College of Rheumatology (ACR) strongly recommends that patients with hip or knee OA participate in aerobic and/or resistance exercises, aquatic exercise and, if overweight, a weight-loss program. In its guidelines, the agency gave conditional recommendations for the use of acetaminophen, nonsteroidal anti-inflammatory drugs (NSAIDs), tramadol (Ultram), and corticosteroid injections, and noted that opioid analgesics should be reserved only for patients who are candidates for joint replacement but can't (or choose not to) have the surgery. The ACR gave a conditional recommendation that knee OA patients be treated with topical NSAIDs (especially those over age 75), viscosupplementation, tai chi, acupuncture, or transcutaneous electrical nerve stimulation (TENS). The group also conditionally recommended against the use of glucosamine or chondroitin supplements for either hip or knee OA, and against using topical capsaicin for knee OA (see Chapter 5 for more on alternative therapies).

For hand OA, the ACR conditionally recommended that doctors evaluate patients' abilities to perform activities of daily living, instruct them on the use of splints for thumb arthritis, and consider treatment with topical capsaicin or topical NSAIDs, oral NSAIDs, and/or tramadol.

Exercise is a key part of a total treatment program for knee OA, as outlined in guidelines from the American Academy of Orthopaedic Surgeons (AAOS). The organization advocates weight loss of five percent of body weight for overweight patients, and the use of NSAIDs or tramadol for patients with symptomatic knee OA, unless they have contraindications. The AAOS did not recommend the use of hyaluronic acid injections (viscosupplementation), acupuncture, glucosamine and/or chondroitin supplements, custom lateral-wedge shoe insoles, or needle lavage (cleaning of the knee joint with saline) for treating knee OA, and advised against arthroscopic lavage of the knee in patients with only symptoms of OA and no other problems, such as a torn meniscus. The AAOS did not recommend for or against the use of the following: acetaminophen, opioids, or pain patches; electrotherapeutic treatments, such as ultrasound or TENS; braces; injections of intra-articular corticosteroids, growth factors, and/or platelet-rich-plasma; or manual therapy (e.g. joint manipulation or chiropractic).

BOX 1-6

OA symptoms

In addition to the common symptoms listed on the previous page and at right, people with OA can have the following symptoms:

- Bony growths: OA can cause bony growths or nodes (Heberden's nodes) to develop in the joints at the ends of the fingers. These growths are not always painful.

- Instability: In some joints, such as the knee, the ligaments that support the joint stretch, and the joint becomes unstable.

- Inflammation: Studies have shown that inflammation of the joint lining (synovitis), which more often occurs in RA, is more common in OA than was previously thought. This inflammation contributes to cartilage degradation, the hallmark characteristic of OA, and may contribute to heightened pain sensitivity.

BOX 1-7

Treat-to-target approach may lower RA mortality risk

Rheumatoid arthritis (RA) increases the risk of premature death, but early aggressive treatment aiming for a goal of low RA disease activity may reduce this mortality risk, recent evidence suggests. For 10 years, Dutch researchers used this tight treat-to-target strategy on 508 patients with recent-onset RA. The patients were divided into four different treatment arms, and medication adjustments were made to achieve a low disease activity as measured by using the Disease Activity Score (DAS). They compared the survival rates of these patients to that of the general Dutch population. During that period, 72 of the participants died, at an average age of 75, and no survival differences were seen between the treatment strategies. The study authors concluded that the treat-to-target approach reduced the mortality rate among the RA patients to a rate comparable to the general Dutch population.

American College of Rheumatology Annual Meeting, November 2014

RA: Treatment goals and strategies

With rheumatoid arthritis (RA), in which symptoms can flare up and then disappear for extended periods of time, early diagnosis is often challenging. Yet it is crucial to begin treatment before the joint becomes seriously damaged. Evidence suggests a "window of opportunity" in early RA and that hitting the disease early and hard with combinations of disease-modifying drugs during this window can push arthritis into remission, or minimize joint damage. For instance, in a study published in the February 2015 issue of *Annals of the Rheumatic Diseases*, Norwegian researchers concluded that the initiation of more aggressive treatment strategies between 2000 and 2010 resulted in a more than twofold increase in the number of patients who achieved RA remission at six months.

A number of experts have adopted a "treat-to-target" strategy—similar to that used in diabetes management—in which RA patients are evaluated frequently and treated aggressively until they reach a state of low disease activity or remission. This strategy may reduce the elevated risk of death associated with RA, a recent study suggests (see Box 1-7, "Treat-to-target approach may lower RA mortality risk").

The immediate treatment goal for RA is to reduce joint inflammation. Caught early enough, RA can often be managed with medications, avoiding the need for surgery. Evidence suggests that doctors and patients are doing just that, as rates of joint-replacement surgery related to RA appear to be on the decline. And today, patients with RA also are enjoying better quality of life than they did in years past. A 2014 study found that in the last two decades, the level of psychological distress and physical disability experienced by RA patients has decreased significantly.

DIAGNOSING ARTHRITIS

Prompt diagnosis of arthritis, especially rheumatoid arthritis (RA), is critical so that treatment can be started to ease pain and minimize damage to cartilage, bone, and ligaments. A careful review of your medical history, a thorough physical examination, and imaging and laboratory tests can determine the type of arthritis you have and the type of treatment you need.

The medical history

Carefully document your symptoms—including the duration, location, and pattern of your pain—and share this information with your physician. Your doctor will inquire about your personal and family medical history. See box 2-1, "Common questions," for a list of possible questions.

▶ Morning stiffness: Another hallmark of both rheumatoid arthritis (RA) and osteoarthritis (OA) is morning stiffness. For those with OA, the temporary stiffness in the back, hips, and other joints usually subsides within a half-hour or so. For those with RA, the stiffness may require several hours, if not all morning, to finally clear. People with RA who sit in one place too long are also more likely to become stiff.

▶ Exercise and rest: RA can often be distinguished from OA on the basis of how joint pain responds to activity and to rest. OA pain tends to gradually worsen if you're on your feet all day, but then eases at night with rest. However, RA joint pain and stiffness may ease when you stand up and move about, but may not be relieved by bed rest.

▶ Steady or episodic pain: Whether your joint pain is steady or comes and goes is another measure used to help distinguish between the two forms of arthritis. OA results in continuous pain that gradually worsens over time. Conversely, RA can be episodic or constant, alternating between painful flare-ups that last for days or weeks, and months of less pain or even remission.

OA tends to be characterized by the slow, steady breakdown of joint cartilage, and results in continuous pain that gradually worsens over time. RA is less predictable, and can be episodic or constant.

BOX 2-1

Common questions:

- Is the pain in one or more joints?
- When does the pain occur?
- How long does the pain last?
- When did you first notice the pain?
- What were you doing when you first noticed the pain?
- Have you had any illnesses or accidents that may account for the pain?
- What medications are you taking?
- Does activity make the pain better or worse?
- Is there a family history of any arthritis or other rheumatic disease?

BOX 2-2

How OA and RA compare

OSTEOARTHRITIS (OA)	RHEUMATOID ARTHRITIS (RA)
DEFINITION	
Disease of the cartilage; related to mechanical stress.	Disease of the joint lining; related to faulty immune system.
LOCATION	
Common in knees, hips, and spine, sometimes in outer finger joints (fingertips and thumb). May not be symmetrical.	Common in hands, wrists, and fingers. Begins in base joints. Affects both sides of the body equally. Often affects joints such as elbows, shoulders, knees, hips, ankles, and toes.
AGE	
Common in people over age 60.	Peak onset is between ages 30 and 50, but can occur at any age.
SEX	
Equally common in men and women, but develops earlier in men.	Three times more common in women than men.
MORNING STIFFNESS	
Lasts less than 20 minutes.	May last several hours or more.
PAIN PROFILE	
Pain worsens with joint use, eases with rest. Gets gradually worse over time.	Pain variable, may disrupt sleep. Stiffness may ease with use. Can flare up, then recede for weeks at a time.
X-RAY PROFILE	
Irregular narrowing of joint space with random bony outgrowths.	Symmetrical erosions and thinning of bone.
BLOOD MARKERS	
No clinically established markers yet.	Probable diagnosis made on basis of rheumatoid factor, cyclic citrullinated peptide (CCP, see page 19), and markers for inflammation.

The physical exam

In the physical exam, your doctor will examine your painful joints, looking for tenderness, redness, warmth, or a buildup of fluid, as well as to get a sense of any limited motion, deformity, or instability. If RA is suspected, the distribution of inflammation is important in making the diagnosis, since in this disease the hands, wrists, feet, and knees are typically inflamed symmetrically (see Box 2-2, "How OA and RA compare").

It's in the hands…

When your hands are affected by either RA or OA, your doctor will look to the pattern of finger involvement to help distinguish the two. RA occurs more often in the joints at the base of your fingers (the metacarpal-phalangeal joints, or MCPs) and the joints in the middle of the fingers (the proximal interphalangeal joints, or PIPs. OA is more common in the base of the thumbs (the first carpometacarpal joints), and the knuckles at the end and middle of your fingers (the distal interphalangeal joints and the PIPs). This difference is so marked that your doctor may apply gentle pressure across the MCPs to evaluate for swelling and tenderness. For RA, the diagnosis often involves the hand and/or wrist joints. More than 90 percent of patients with RA have the disease in the base of their fingers, near the knuckles. For OA, the hand or wrist may or may not be involved.

…Or hips

OA frequently occurs in the large weight-bearing joints of your hips, knees, and spine. Conversely, RA usually occurs first in the smaller joints of your hands, and the wrists.

Radiological imaging
X-rays

X-rays remain the most important imaging method for determining the severity of your arthritis. Though X-rays show only the position of the bones, the space between bones is an accurate reflection of how much healthy cartilage remains. Narrowing of this space over time is associated with loss of cartilage and can be used to monitor the further advance of OA and RA.

OA and RA look quite different on X-rays. With RA, small

erosions or destruction of the bone can be seen, as well as thinning of the bones around the joints (periarticular osteopenia). With OA, you will see tiny irregular outgrowths or bone spurs (osteophytes).

MRI/magnetic resonance imaging

Since X-ray evidence for RA may not be apparent until you have the disease for six to 12 months or longer, physicians are turning to magnetic resonance imaging (MRI) to help with earlier detection. Some evidence suggests that MRI may detect inflammation in joints without any apparent clinical inflammation in patients with early RA.

An MRI helps the doctor evaluate the soft tissues in and around a joint that are not visible on X-ray, including ligaments, tendons, and the crescent-shaped pieces of cartilage (the menisci) that partly cover the ends of your knee bones. Conventional MRIs assess cartilage quality in people with joint pain or diagnosed arthritis. Newer, more advanced MRI techniques can detect subtle changes in cartilage that may indicate early OA and allow for earlier treatment.

Ultrasound

Due to its low cost, absence of radiation and speed of imaging, ultrasonography is an attractive method of imaging. Compared to standard X-rays, ultrasound may be more effective at detecting early-stage bone erosion.

Laboratory tests
Osteoarthritis: Lab tests may be ahead

Though there are no current blood tests to confirm the presence of OA, several are being investigated. Researchers are studying certain blood biomarkers, micro RNAs, that may predict which patients will develop OA that necessitates joint-replacement surgery. Other investigations focus on proteins known as galectins, which trigger degenerative and inflammatory responses in cartilage cells and may play a significant role in OA.

Overall, experts have identified a number of biomarkers, including markers of collagen synthesis and degradation that signify cartilage breakdown, as well as markers of bone and synovium breakdown.

Rheumatoid arthritis: Lab tests for inflammation

Complete blood count (CBC)

A complete blood count measures the amount of red blood cells, white blood cells, and platelets in your blood, as well as other key blood levels.

- An elevated white blood cell count may suggest inflammation due to RA. However, other conditions, such as an infection or a cold, can cause a similar spike in the count.
- A low red blood cell count (low hematocrit) often indicates an iron deficiency or an anemia of chronic disease. Since 50 percent of people with RA have such anemia, it adds to the circumstantial evidence for RA.
- Increased platelets can also be present when there is systemic inflammation.

Comprehensive Metabolic Panel (CMP)

- A blood chemistry screen can also help identify damage to other organs, such as the kidneys, which may be affected by RA.
- It is important to get baseline liver function tests prior to starting RA medications. Liver enzymes can also be elevated in chronic hepatitis B or C, which can cause an inflammatory arthritis similar to RA.

Erythrocyte sedimentation rate (ESR)

When inflammation is present, your body makes proteins that cause your red blood cells (erythrocytes) to clump. Since clumped cells fall out of solution faster than unclumped ones, measuring the rate of this fall (or sedimentation) gives a rough indication of the level of inflammation present.

C-reactive protein (CRP)

Levels of this protein may increase in those with RA and may decrease when NSAIDs or corticosteroids are used to reduce inflammation.

Other inflammatory markers

Researchers continue to examine other markers of inflammation that may signal RA risk. Among these are soluble tumor necrosis factor receptor II and interleukin-6, which are increased in people with active RA, sometimes years before they develop symptoms.

Some research suggests these markers may accurately predict which patients will develop active RA.

Rheumatoid arthritis: Lab tests for marker proteins

Rheumatoid factor

About 80 percent of people with RA have this immune system protein (antibody) in their blood. However, rheumatoid factor is present in people with other connective tissue disorders, such as systemic lupus erythematosus, with infectious diseases such as syphilis, mononucleosis or hepatitis, and in those with liver disease. It may even be found in healthy people, particularly if a person has a close relative with RA.

Antinuclear antibody (ANA)

Approximately one-half of those with RA will have this protein in their blood.

Anti-CCP (antibodies to cyclic citrullinated peptide)

This test for citrulline antibodies is a valuable tool in the early diagnosis of RA, especially among people deemed at higher risk for the disease. Studies show that CCP antibodies may be detected in the blood up to 10 years before a patient shows symptoms of RA. When the antibody is detected in the blood, you have a 90 to 95 percent likelihood of having RA. A 2014 study found that a risk score using anti-CCP and other factors could accurately predict a person's risk of progressing to RA.

Markers under study

Researchers reported in 2014 that a protein known as serum 14-3-3-eta distinguished people with RA from healthy patients and those with other autoimmune disorders or OA, with capabilities comparable to rheumatoid factor and anti-CCP. Serum 14-3-3-eta was associated with more severe RA and also enhanced the detection of the disease when combined with rheumatoid factor and anti-CCP, the study found.

Scientists also have discovered that in the most severe cases of RA, the immune system creates a unique set of disease-promoting antibodies, such as antibodies to peptidylarginine deiminase 4 (PAD4). In one study, 80 percent of patients with these antibodies

Hand OA linked to cardiac risks

Recent research suggests that people with symptomatic hand osteoarthritis (OA) may face an increased risk of cardiac complications. In the study, researchers reviewed data on 1,348 participants (average age about 62) in the Framingham Heart Study, including 726 with evidence of hand OA based on symptoms or radiographic (X-ray) imaging. The researchers found that those with symptomatic hand OA, but not radiographic OA alone, were at increased risk of heart attack or coronary insufficiency (inadequate blood flow in the coronary arteries).

Annals of the Rheumatic Diseases, January 2015

Drugs may reduce cardiovascular risks in RA patients

Treating rheumatoid arthritis (RA) with the drug hydroxychloroquine (Plaquenil) may lower cardiovascular morbidity, while treatment with tumor necrosis factor (TNF) inhibitors does not increase the risk of heart failure and may even protect against it, two recent studies suggest. In the first study, researchers found that among 514 RA patients, use of hydroxychloroquine (especially at the higher standard dose of 400 mg a day) reduced the risk of heart attack, stroke, and other cardiovascular events, compared to non-use. In the second study, researchers noted that TNF inhibitors have been associated with worsening of existing heart failure. But, after reviewing data on more than 16,000 RA patients, they found a reduced risk of new heart failure among those on anti-TNF therapy, compared to patients treated with non-biologic disease-modifying antirheumatic drugs, such as methotrexate.

American College of Rheumatology Annual Meeting, November 2014

experienced a worsening of their RA in the previous year, compared to 53 percent of those without the antibodies.

Complications beyond the joints
Arthritis: Cardiovascular assessment

Research has shown that people with RA are at increased risk for cardiovascular disease. In fact, evidence suggests that the cardiovascular risk posed by RA is comparable to that of a leading cardiovascular disease risk factor, diabetes.

Studies suggest that the risk of heart attack nearly doubles within the first 10 years of an RA diagnosis, and people with the disease suffer greater complications after a heart attack. The inflammation associated with RA may contribute to atherosclerosis, or "hardening" of the arteries. Other evidence ties RA to an increased risk of the most common irregular heart rhythm, atrial fibrillation, which is a leading stroke risk factor. RA patients are at greater risk of another cardiac condition, heart failure, and they also face a higher risk of venous thromboembolism, a blood clot that forms within a vein and may cause a life-threatening pulmonary embolism.

An osteoarthritis-cardiovascular connection?

While RA is a well-established cardiovascular risk factor, the effects of OA on heart health are not so well elucidated. One study found that people with OA were at greater risk of cardiovascular problems, especially those with severe OA requiring joint replacement. Another found that people with symptomatic hand OA faced increased cardiovascular risks (see Box 2-3, "Hand OA linked to cardiac risks"). Researchers haven't identified a mechanism underlying a potential OA-cardiovascular connection. One explanation could be that people with symptomatic OA tend to be on treatment with nonsteroidal anti-inflammatory medications, which have been associated with increased cardiovascular risk. Another potential reason is that disability caused by OA results in physical inactivity and being overweight, raising the risk for diabetes and heart disease. In a 2015 study, published in *Annals of the Rheumatic Diseases*, investigators found no link between OA and greater cardiovascular risk among 4,648 people who were followed an average of more than 14 years. However, people with increasing disability were more likely to suffer a cardiovascular event, independent of the presence of OA.

Reducing cardiovascular risks

After diagnosing RA, your doctor should screen for cardiovascular risk factors—such as high blood pressure, abnormal cholesterol levels, diabetes, obesity, and smoking—and work with you to manage them and reduce your risk. You may even be referred to a preventive cardiologist for a cardiac risk assessment, using risk-prediction tools that include traditional cardiovascular risk factors as well as RA-specific factors.

Given the serious cardiovascular risks posed by RA, seek prompt treatment for the disease. Evidence suggests that certain drug treatments for RA reduce the risk of cardiovascular events by effectively controlling the disease activity and decreasing inflammation. The best studied are methotrexate, and tumor necrosis factor inhibitors (see Box 2-4, "Drugs may reduce cardiovascular risks in RA patients"). Likewise, it's critical to follow your doctor's advice to lower your cardiovascular risk through lifestyle changes and, if necessary, medications.

Rheumatoid arthritis: Extra-articular manifestations

In addition to its damaging effects on the joints and the cardiovascular system, RA may affect a number of other areas of the body—what experts refer to as extra-articular manifestations—including the lungs (see Box 2-5, "Women with RA more likely to die from respiratory and other causes"). RA may cause painful breathing, shortness of breath, scarring of the lungs, and lung nodules. In some cases, RA-related lung problems can develop before joint symptoms. Additionally, the incidence of chronic obstructive pulmonary disease (COPD) in people with RA is double that of those without the disease. So, have your respiratory health monitored, and seek an evaluation if you experience breathing difficulties, such as shortness of breath, chronic coughing, and chest tightness.

People with RA also should be aware of potential kidney disorders and gastrointestinal (GI) problems. A 2014 study found that people with RA have a one in four chance of developing chronic kidney disease, compared to a one in five chance among those

Women with RA more likely to die from respiratory and other causes

Women with rheumatoid arthritis (RA) face a significantly greater risk of death from all causes, especially respiratory problems, according to a recent study. Among 121,700 women followed for 34 years, 960 had RA and 25,699 died, including 261 deaths among the RA patients. The researchers calculated that the risk of death from any cause was twofold higher among women with RA compared to their RA-free counterparts. More specifically, the risk of death from respiratory causes was 4.5 times greater among women with RA versus those without RA, the study found.

American College of Rheumatology Annual Meeting, November 2014

without RA. Other evidence suggests that RA patients may be more likely to develop GI disorders such as stomach ulcers, bleeding, infectious colitis, and diverticulitis.

RA can manifest in the skin as nodules or rashes, and it can cause peripheral neuropathy, nerve damage characterized by numbness, tingling, or burning pain. It commonly causes poor sleep and fatigue. The pain and difficulties associated with the disease also can lead to depression and anxiety, and some evidence has linked depression with slower improvement in RA disease activity. So, report any depressive symptoms (such as feelings of sadness and hopelessness, trouble focusing, and a lack of pleasure from things you used to enjoy) to your doctor.

Another common consequence of RA is osteoporosis, a loss of bone mass that increases your risk of fractures. Compounding the problem is that RA patients (and arthritis patients in general) are at a greater risk of falls and fall-related injuries. As such, your doctor may discuss fall-prevention strategies, and suggest that you undergo bone-density testing every two years to assess your bone health.

Some patients with RA develop ocular (eye) complications, such as dry eye, inflammation of the blood vessels in the white of the eye (scleritis), and inflammation of the iris (iritis, or anterior uveitis). If you have RA and no eye symptoms, your doctor may suggest you see your eye specialist for an exam every year or two after age 40. If you develop pain, severe redness, or light sensitivity, consult an ophthalmologist.

Other tests/procedures
Lab tests that look for signs in the joint fluid
If fluid has accumulated in a joint, your doctor may remove some with a needle in a procedure called aspiration, and have it examined. The fluid can be tested for signs of increased inflammation that would be seen with RA, or it can detect any evidence of infection. Analysis of the fluid can also help rule out gout, a form of inflammatory arthritis.

Arthroscopy
This is a minimally invasive surgical procedure in which a doctor looks for joint damage by using an arthroscope, a small camera

that is inserted through a 1 cm incision into the joint space. Used most frequently on the knee, the procedure lets a doctor examine the internal structures and check for damage to ligaments, cartilage, or menisci that may be treated arthroscopically.

Putting it all together

RA can be difficult to identify in its earliest stages. No single test can be used to diagnose the disease, and its symptoms and their severity can differ from person to person. Also, because symptoms can be similar to those of other types of arthritis and joint problems, it may take time to rule out those other conditions.

The American College of Rheumatology and the European League Against Rheumatism define a diagnosis of "definite" RA as:

▶ **Confirmed presence of joint swelling,** indicating synovitis—inflammation of the synovial membrane that lines the joint—in at least one joint.

▶ **Absence of an alternative diagnosis** that might better explain the symptoms (synovitis), such as gout or lupus.

▶ **A combined score of six or higher** (out of a possible 10) from the following tests/investigations:

  • number and sites of affected joints
  • blood test results (for autoantibodies indicative of RA)
  • increase in inflammatory proteins, and
  • duration of symptoms.

MEDICATIONS THAT TREAT PAIN AND INFLAMMATION

Prescription and over-the-counter medications are a cornerstone of arthritis treatment, providing relief of pain and inflammation. The broad array of oral, topical, injectable, and infusible drugs vary in their mechanism of action and their effectiveness. And, like all medications, arthritis drugs are associated with a range of side effects, some only bothersome but others potentially more harmful. So, whether you have osteoarthritis (OA) or rheumatoid arthritis (RA), it's important to understand the pros and cons of the medications you take and to review their risks and benefits with your physician.

Broad categories of arthritis drugs
First-line, fast-acting drugs
These take effect in hours or days and are used widely to treat pain and inflammation for both OA and RA. They include aspirin, ibuprofen (Advil, Motrin), naproxen (Aleve, Naprosyn), and other nonsteroidal anti-inflammatory drugs (NSAIDs), and acetaminophen (Tylenol). Corticosteroids, such as prednisone (Deltasone, Cortan, Sterapred), are also used as fast-acting relief for RA patients.

Oral pain relievers and analgesics:
- Acetaminophen
- Corticosteroids
- NSAIDs

Second-line, slower-acting drugs for rheumatoid arthritis
Disease-modifying antirheumatic drugs, or DMARDs, are slower-acting than first-line medications but often more effective. Because DMARDs take weeks or months to take effect, they are used in combination with faster-acting first-line drugs. DMARDS have more potent side effects, and their use should be carefully monitored.

DMARDs:
- Hydroxychloroquine (Plaquenil)
- Leflunomide (Arava)
- Methotrexate (Rheumatrex)
- Sulfasalazine (Azulfidine)

Third-line, immune system-modifying drugs

These drugs slow down the inflammatory process by interfering with specific chemical messengers of the immune system. These are the most potent of all RA medications and among the most expensive, with equally powerful side effects that need to be carefully monitored. These drugs are used if traditional therapy from first- and second-line drugs fails to adequately control the progression of RA.

Biological response modifiers:

- Adalimumab (Humira)
- Anakinra (Kineret)
- Certolizumab (Cimzia)
- Etanercept (Enbrel)
- Golimumab (Simponi)
- Infliximab (Remicade)
- Tocilizumab (Actemra)
- Tofacitinib (Xeljanz)

Cell blockers:

- Abatacept (Orencia)
- Rituximab (Rituxan)

First-line, fast-acting drugs
Analgesics & anti-inflammatories

This is a broad category of medications that includes over-the-counter drugs for pain relief, such as acetaminophen (Tylenol), as well as those that fight pain and inflammation.

Because analgesics are often non-prescription and widely available, it's easy to assume they are completely safe. However, they contain some of the same ingredients found in prescription medications, and they can have side effects, reacting with other medicines or supplements you're taking. Be careful when taking several of these at once, since you can end up taking a larger combined dose of a particular drug than you realize. When buying any over-the-counter pain relievers, read labels carefully, focusing on the list of active ingredients and dosages. Make sure your comparisons are of drugs with the same active ingredient. If you start taking a prescription analgesic or anti-inflammatory, stop taking over-the-counter versions. If you don't, you magnify the risk of side effects.

Acetaminophen

Acetaminophen (Tylenol) eases pain by acting on the part of your brain that receives the pain signals. Though it doesn't help with

Acetaminophen ineffective for back pain

The popular pain reliever acetaminophen (Tylenol) has no effect on low back pain, and is of limited short-term benefit for relieving knee or hip osteoarthritis (OA) pain, a recent meta-analysis suggests. Researchers reviewing data from 13 randomized, controlled studies involving more than 5,300 people found that acetaminophen did not ease low-back pain, reduce disability, or improve quality of life. The drug fared somewhat better at reducing pain and disability from hip and knee OA, but the improvements were not clinically significant. Additionally, compared to those given a placebo, acetaminophen users were four times more likely to have abnormal results on liver function tests.

British Medical Journal, April 2015

inflammation, acetaminophen generally does help you avoid the bleeding problems and gastrointestinal side effects associated with NSAIDs. Although many experts recommend acetaminophen as a first-line pain reliever, a 2015 study questioned its efficacy (see Box 3-1, "Acetaminophen ineffective for back pain").

Acetaminophen appears to be safe for long-term use, as long as you don't have a liver weakened by alcohol use or other diseases, or take too much of the drug. Problems arise when people overdose by using multiple products containing acetaminophen, ranging from over-the-counter painkillers and cold medicines to some prescription pain medicines. The liver breaks down acetaminophen, and taking too much puts excess stress on that organ. Take no more than 3,000 milligrams (mg)—about six extra-strength pills—of acetaminophen a day. In 2014, the U.S. Food and Drug Administration (FDA) ordered all makers of prescription combination drugs containing acetaminophen to limit the acetaminophen content in these products to 325 mg or less.

Check all your labels carefully to determine just how much of this drug you might be taking—more than 600 products, including several NSAIDs, contain acetaminophen. (Look on your prescription bottles for the abbreviation "APAP," used by many doctors and pharmacists to identify acetaminophen.) And if you regularly use alcohol or have a weakened liver, discuss this with your doctor before taking acetaminophen.

NSAIDs

NSAIDs relieve the pain and inflammation of a variety of conditions, including arthritis. They are considered first-line drugs (see Box 3-2, "Nonsteroidal anti-inflammatory drugs [NSAIDs]"). Low doses of NSAIDs may be enough for OA, but a doctor will often prescribe higher doses for RA because of more severe swelling, redness, and joint stiffness. Combinations of two or more NSAIDs should generally be avoided, since they are no more effective when used together and may have additive side effects.

You are at greater risk of stomach irritation from NSAID use if you:

- Have pre-existing ulcers (stomach inflammation, peptic ulcers)
- Smoke cigarettes
- Are in poor general health

- Are taking prednisone or cortisone
- Are over age 60
- Are taking NSAIDs for an extended period of time.

COX-2 inhibitors

A member of a class of NSAIDs known as COX-2 inhibitors, celecoxib (Celebrex) relieves pain and inflammation but, unlike traditional NSAIDs, is less likely to irritate your stomach.

NSAID warnings

The benefits of NSAIDs, particularly COX-2 inhibitors, have been overshadowed somewhat by evidence that these popular drugs pose a cardiovascular risk, especially to those with pre-existing heart disease. Two COX-2 medications—rofecoxib (Vioxx) and valdecoxib (Bextra)—were removed from U.S. and European markets after being linked with increased risks of heart attack and stroke. Celebrex remains the only COX-2 painkiller available, although it's still the subject of controversy and it carries a black box warning about increased cardiovascular risk. The American Heart Association recommends that COX-2 drugs be used only as a last resort in people with or at high risk of cardiovascular disease, and in the lowest dose and for the shortest duration necessary.

Though over-the-counter NSAIDs such as ibuprofen (Advil, Motrin) and naproxen (Aleve, Naprosyn) pose less cardiac risk than COX-2 drugs, research suggests that these commonly used painkillers may still increase your risk of heart attack, especially if you have a history of heart attack, take high doses, or use the drugs frequently and over an extended period of time.

The overall evidence suggests that NSAIDs (but not aspirin) may raise the risk of heart attack, stroke, and other cardiovascular events. The drugs may increase blood pressure, and reduce the effects of some blood pressure medications. NSAIDs and high-dose aspirin also may have adverse effects on the kidneys, and generally should be avoided in people with decreased renal function. Additionally, use of NSAIDs is associated with a greater risk of gastrointestinal complications, such as stomach ulcers and gastrointestinal (GI) bleeding.

The FDA has mandated the following labeling requirements for all NSAIDs:

BOX 3-2

Nonsteroidal anti-inflammatory drugs (NSAIDs)	
GENERIC NAME	BRAND NAME(S)
aspirin*	Anacin, Ascriptin, Bayer, Bufferin, Ecotrin, Excedrin
diclofenac	Cambia, Cataflam, Voltaren, Zipsor, Zorvolex
etodolac	Lodine
ibuprofen	Advil, Motrin
indomethacin	Indocin
ketoprofen	
meloxicam	Mobic
naproxen	Aleve, Naprosyn
piroxicam	Feldene

*Active ingredient: salicylate

BOX 3-3

Six ways to save on drug costs

- **Split pills:** Ask your doctor to prescribe your pills in double strength. Then, using a plastic pill-cutter, split them in half. Note: Medications such as time-release pills, capsules, and tablets coated to reduce stomach irritation lose their effectiveness when split.

- **Buy generics:** Once a patent runs out on a well-known drug, others made of the same chemicals hit the market with a different name at a lower price. Ask your doctor if there's a generic version of your pain medication.

- **Stick with the tried and true:** The newest pain medication is not always more effective than your current one, but it will cost more. Stick with the older, cheaper drug unless your doctor believes the newer one is significantly more effective.

- **Consider an alternative drug:** Arthritis pain, like most conditions, can be effectively managed by a variety of medications. Ask about other drugs that may be priced lower but have the same effect.

- **Take more often:** Generally, pills that must be taken two or three times a day are less expensive than those made to be taken only once a day. However, taking more pills will require you to be more disciplined and may not be for you if you're likely to forget to take your next dose.

- **Shop for better prices:** Compare prices at online pharmacies. The National Association of Boards of Pharmacy offers a list of approved online pharmacies at www.awarerx.org. Also, check senior discounts. Most pharmacies offer some sort of discount for seniors, but shop around, since it can vary from a flat sum to as high as 60 percent for some medications.

▶ **Prescription NSAIDs:** These drugs include a black box warning that highlights the potential increased risk for heart attack and stroke, as well as potentially life-threatening GI bleeding.

▶ **Over-the-counter NSAIDs (except aspirin):** Labeling includes specific information about the potential for GI and cardiovascular side effects, a reminder to follow label instructions, and a warning about potential skin reactions.

▶ **Less is more:** All NSAIDs should be prescribed at the lowest effective dose for the shortest duration consistent with individual treatment goals.

Some evidence suggests different degrees of cardiovascular safety among the NSAIDs. In particular, some studies have concluded that naproxen may have a safer cardiovascular risk profile, prompting calls to remove the warning about cardiovascular side effects from naproxen products. However, in 2014, an FDA advisory panel recommended that the label warning remain, determining that available evidence is insufficient to prove conclusively that naproxen is safer on the heart.

Experts hope that an ongoing clinical trial, PRECISION, will provide more definitive answers about the safety of NSAIDs. The study, led by Cleveland Clinic, is assessing the cardiovascular risks of celecoxib, ibuprofen, and naproxen among 20,000 arthritis patients with or at risk of developing cardiovascular disease.

Despite the safety concerns about NSAIDs, one study, involving 923 patients followed for an average of more than 10 years, found that people with RA in multiple joints who took NSAIDs did not have an increased risk of dying. In fact, NSAID use was associated with a reduced risk of heart-related death, the study found.

A note on drug costs

Arthritis pain relievers, including NSAIDs, can be expensive. However, talk to your doctor about ways you can get the most out of your pills and cut your costs (see Box 3-3, "Six ways to save on drug costs").

Strategies for managing your NSAID use

With the warnings about risks from prescription and traditional NSAIDs, you now have to work harder to find new strategies for managing your arthritis pain. Here are some options to consider:

- **NSAIDs might be avoided altogether:** Fully pursue non-drug options, such as exercise to strengthen the muscles around the joint, use of topical analgesics, and weight loss. The more you can use these to relieve pain, the lower the dose of NSAIDs you may need.

- **Analgesics may be enough:** If your arthritis involves little or no inflammation, a simple analgesic, such as acetaminophen (Tylenol, Excedrin), rather than an NSAID, may provide enough pain relief.

- **Try low-cost,** over-the-counter NSAIDs first: These include ibuprofen (Advil, Motrin) and naproxen (Aleve). Your doctor might have you try one of these alone or in combination with an analgesic. You may need to try several of them before finding one that provides your best combination of pain relief, inflammation control, and minimal side effects.

- **Use prescription-strength NSAIDs only when necessary,** when over-the-counter, traditional NSAIDs don't provide you with sufficient pain relief.

Steps for minimizing stomach irritation

As traditional NSAIDs possibly become a bigger part of your pain-management strategy, you'll need increased efforts to deal with the risk of stomach irritation. Here are some options to help minimize such risk:

- **Always take an NSAID with food,** and take only one type at a time.

- **Reduce aspirin dose or frequency.** The key to avoiding side effects is in the dosage; one baby aspirin (80 mg per day) or one adult aspirin (325 mg every other day) makes side effects less likely. Taking coated aspirin, which are a bit more expensive, also may lower the risk.

- **To help relieve stomach irritation,** your doctor may suggest a histamine (H2) blocker, such as cimetidine (Tagamet) and ranitidine (Zantac), which decrease stomach acid production.

- **To help reduce the amount of stomach acid you produce,** your doctor may prescribe an NSAID in combination with a type of medicine called a proton pump inhibitor, such as esomeprazole (Nexium) or omeprazole (Prilosec).

- **Another option is to combine your NSAID with misoprostol (Cytotec),** a drug that puts back the stomach-protecting prostaglandins

Steroid injections may hurt your hips

Steroid injections are commonly used to manage the pain and inflammation of hip osteoarthritis, but two recent studies raise concerns about the shots. One study found that within six months of receiving ultrasound-guided intra-articular hip injections with the corticosteroid triamcinolone acetate and lidocaine, all but one of 33 patients showed decreases in joint space width (a sign of advancing arthritis visible on X-ray). Another study showed that intra-articular cortico-steroids have a "profound" dose-dependent impact on cells found in bone marrow, suggesting that the injections increase the progression of joint disease. While some hip degeneration due to arthritis is natural, steroid injections were associated with more rapid progression of severe bone loss and partial dislocation of the joint, the researchers stated.

American Academy of Orthopaedic Surgeons Annual Meeting, March 2015

---

that aspirin and other traditional NSAIDs take away. This synthetic prostaglandin is designed to help heal existing ulcers and reduce the risk of new ones.

Corticosteroids: A more potent analgesic and anti-inflammatory option

Steroid injections for osteoarthritis

When the inflammation and pain are limited largely to one joint, as is often the case with OA, injections of corticosteroid medication into the joint space may be helpful; however, the effectiveness can vary by joint type. A 2014 study found that adding a corticosteroid to epidural injections of lidocaine provided no significant additional benefit over lidocaine alone for treating pain and disability from spinal stenosis. Additionally, research suggests that overuse of cortisone may damage or weaken cartilage and tendons near the joint, and, over time, corticosteroids may reduce bone density and increase fracture risk (see Box 3-4, "Steroid injections may hurt your hips"). So, many experts recommend limiting the injections to no more than three times a year and no more than 10 times per joint in a patient's lifetime; however, this depends on the joint being injected and on each patient's individual circumstances.

Corticosteroids for rheumatoid arthritis

Corticosteroids, either as pill or injection, can provide quick relief from flare-ups of RA pain and inflammation. But because of added risk to cartilage health if used too often, corticosteroids are used only to treat severe flare-ups or buy time until the slower-acting DMARDs take effect, and are then discontinued. While they work very well for pain and inflammation, their long-term use is associated with several potential adverse affects. These include increased infection risk, weight gain, diabetes, osteoporosis, cata-racts, glaucoma, hypertension, stomach ulcers, easy bruising, and mood changes, among others. Therefore they are used at the lowest dose possible to control symptoms, with the goal of stop-ping them completely as other DMARDs take effect.

Codeine and other narcotics: Heavy-duty pain relief

If anti-inflammatory drugs fail to blunt your arthritis pain, your doctor may suggest more powerful pain medications, such as those with codeine or opiate-containing narcotics (opioids). Examples are hydrocodone (Lortab, Norco), oxycodone (OxyContin, Percocet), and the synthetic opioid tramadol (Ultram).

While effective, opioids may cause an addiction-like dependence on the drugs, although a review of 26 studies comprising nearly 5,000 patients concluded that long-term use of opioid medications in the right patients carried little risk of addiction. Patients also may develop tolerance to opioids and require higher doses to maintain the same analgesic effects, leading to greater risk of side effects, such as constipation, dizziness, or drowsiness. One study found that opioid use was associated with an increased risk of atrial fibrillation, the most common abnormal heart rhythm and a major risk factor for stroke (see Box 3-5, "Opioids linked to abnormal heart rhythm"). In 2014, the American Academy of Neurology noted in a position statement that the risks associated with opioids outweigh the benefits when the drugs are prescribed for chronic non-cancer pain.

Topical analgesics

Topical analgesics are pain-relief medications that you rub into the skin near the source of pain. Most are available over the counter, without a prescription. Some merely distract you from the underlying pain by creating sensations of heat or coolness, while others actually help block the transmission of pain signals.

Counterirritants

Topical applications that distract you from the pain are known as counterirritants, and they depend largely on menthol, camphor, or methyl salicylate for their temporary effects. Those with menthol or camphor create a cooling sensation; those with methyl salicylate, a feeling of warmth.

Capsaicin creams

These topical creams, made from the active ingredient in hot peppers, have shown some evidence of providing local pain relief for OA. Though not fully understood, it is thought these creams work by interfering with a pain messenger molecule or neurotransmitter (substance P). After a week or more of regular use (three to four times a day), the capsaicin depletes the supply

Opioids linked to abnormal heart rhythm

A large study suggests that use of opioid pain relievers is associated with an increased prevalence of atrial fibrillation (Afib). The study included 24,632 people, average age 65, of whom 1,887 reported opioid use and 2,086 had Afib. The most commonly used opioids were hydrocodone, propoxyphene (removed from the U.S. market in 2010 due to concerns about heart-rhythm abnormalities), and tramadol. The researchers reported that the likelihood of Afib was 35 percent greater in the study participants who used opioids, and that even after propoxyphene users were excluded, the association between opioid use and Afib remained significant.

JAMA Internal Medicine, April 2015

of substance P left in your nerve endings (sensory receptors). Once that happens, they are no longer able to transmit signals of arthritis pain. This benefit will continue as long as you keep using the cream.

Topical NSAIDs

While easing pain, topical NSAIDs may minimize the side effects caused by oral NSAIDs. In the U.S., one prescription product is available—topical diclofenac sodium (Voltaren Gel)—approved specifically for treating OA of the knee, hand, wrist, elbow, ankle, and feet. (A topical diclofenac patch—Flector Patch—is available for treating acute pain from sprains and other injuries.) It is important to let your doctor know about any liver-related problems before using Voltaren Gel or other diclofenac-containing products.

Topical dos and don'ts

Keep in mind that topical analgesics should be seen as temporary relief, not as a long-term solution for your pain.

▶ Topicals are local and site-specific, best used when a single joint hurts, and are not recommended for multi-joint pain, such as with RA.

▶ As with all topical analgesics, but particularly with capsaicin creams and Voltaren Gel, wash your hands immediately after use, and avoid contact with your eyes, nose or mouth.

▶ If you're sensitive to salicylates, or are taking a medication that could interact with salicylates, such as warfarin (Coumadin), use these salves with caution.

On the horizon

Experts are studying another approach to OA pain relief: inhibiting nerve growth factors, which are small proteins released at sites of injury and inflammation. Research has suggested that nerve growth factors appear to accentuate pain, and inhibiting these proteins potentially may offer a new type of therapy to combat OA and other pain conditions.

Some research suggests that injections of tanezumab, a humanized monoclonal antibody that inhibits nerve growth factor, can produce significant improvements in pain, stiffness, and physical function in patients with moderate-to-severe knee

OA, often within days of initial treatment. Despite the positive findings, some patients given the drug as part of a clinical trial developed progressively worsening arthritis, bone degradation, and joint failure that required total joint replacements. In response, the FDA ordered a halting of the clinical research program into tanezumab, but later lifted the ban. So, in 2015 the drug's developer announced plans to resume studies of tanezumab.

OA traditionally has not been considered an inflammatory condition, unlike RA, but research has uncovered higher levels of inflammatory cells in the joints of OA patients. Inflammation contributes to cartilage degradation, the main characteristic of OA. Investigators continue to study drugs like interleukin-1 inhibitors, which target cytokines (proteins that send signals to cells to inflame the joints).

Bone may be to blame

Instead of seeing OA as a problem primarily with cartilage, researchers are examining the interplay between the cartilage and the subchondral bone directly underneath it. In OA, the subchondral bone becomes abnormally thick before cartilage begins to break down. Researchers have found that in mice with anterior cruciate ligament tears (which can lead to knee OA), portions of subchondral bone had been eaten away. Consequently, the mice generated high levels of a protein called TGF-beta1, which, in turn, recruited stem cells to generate new bone to repair the damage. However, the bone-building process overcompensated for the bone damage, stretching the cartilage above and hastening its decline. The researchers noted that this surplus bone formation may be the culprit underlying OA, and that injecting antibodies to TGF-beta1 into the subchondral bone might halt OA progression. Research into this treatment continues.

Second-line, slower-acting drugs
Non-biologic disease-modifying antirheumatic drugs (DMARDs)

These drugs are used to slow the course of RA. Because it often takes a few months before they begin to control swelling, they are typically used in combination with NSAIDs or corticosteroids, which provide short-term relief.

Immunosuppressive drugs

This is a category of DMARDs that hinders the inflammatory response by slowing the reproduction of immune system cells, thereby reducing the amount of enzymes and other chemicals these cells produce. These molecules play a role in stimulating the inflammatory response.

Methotrexate (Rheumatrex, Otrexup)

Methotrexate is the most widely used of these immunosuppressive DMARDs, and is often given for long-term management of RA. More than 50 percent of patients taking methotrexate continue taking it for more than three years, and research suggests it can help people with new-onset RA achieve remission. However, this popular drug, taken orally, doesn't work for everyone, and those who don't tolerate it may be switched to another DMARD or to a self-injectable form (Otrexup). Disadvantages of methotrexate include gastrointestinal side effects (e.g. nausea, vomiting) and the need for ongoing monitoring of liver function and blood counts, to avoid toxicity. In addition, it needs to be stopped three months before a planned pregnancy, as it is toxic to fetuses.

Leflunomide (Arava)

This DMARD has been shown to be about as effective as methotrexate and is sometimes used in combination with the older drug. Clinical trials suggest that leflunomide is safe and effective for up to five years, and can help with long-term management of RA. The most common side effect of this DMARD is diarrhea, which may require the dosage to be lowered or stopped altogether. Other side effects include immunosuppression, birth defects, abdominal pain, rash, and hair loss. Pregnant women or women of childbearing potential who are not using reliable contraception should not use leflunomide, nor should people with pre-existing liver disease or elevated liver enzymes (ALT greater than twice the upper limit of normal). The drug should be used with caution in patients taking other drugs known to cause liver injury.

Hydroxychloroquine

Though this drug is chiefly used to treat malaria, it has also been shown to relieve RA symptoms. Its effects may not be felt for three to six months, and it is not considered a potent immunosuppressive.

Sulfasalazine

This medication doubles as an anti-inflammatory agent and a DMARD, because it not only eases the pain of arthritis, but also may prevent joint damage. Sulfasalazine may be given for mild RA or used in combination with other drugs for people with more severe symptoms. Side effects may include nausea, abdominal discomfort, skin rash, headache, and increased sensitivity to sunlight.

Immunosuppressive drugs/side effects

These medicines can potentially damage blood cells (red blood cells, white blood cells, platelets) and other tissues, so dosages and usage must be carefully monitored. Potential side effects include:

- Anemia: reduced red blood cell count; low iron content.
- Infection risk: lower white blood cell count means fewer cells left to fight off foreign cells and proteins.
- Bleeding risk: fewer platelets mean less ability for blood to clot and halt bleeding.
- Organ damage: methotrexate and leflunomide can damage the liver, and methotrexate can harm the lungs.
- Cancer risk: Some evidence suggests that methotrexate may increase the risk of melanoma, the deadliest form of skin cancer, as well as non-Hodgkin's lymphoma and lung cancer.

The occurrence of side effects depends on the dose, type of medication, and length of treatment. Careful monitoring can minimize these risks.

Third-line, immune system-modifying drugs
Biological response modifiers

This newer category of drugs is reserved for those with moderate-to-severe RA that fails to respond to first- and second-line drugs, like NSAIDs and conventional DMARDs. Medications in this

Methotrexate/biologic combo helps save large joints

RA patients given a combination of methotrexate and either adalimumab or etanercept may be less likely than those given the biologic drugs alone to require replacement of a large joint, according to recent research. The study included 803 RA patients treated with adalimumab or etanercept from 2005 to 2013, including 601 who also were on methotrexate therapy. Forty-nine of the study participants underwent one or more replacements of a large joint (hip, knee, ankle, or elbow). The researchers found that patients given methotrexate in addition to one of the biologic drugs had a significantly lower incidence of large-joint replacement.

Arthritis Care & Research, April 2015

category, also known as immune response modifiers, are genetically engineered to slow down inflammation by interfering with specific chemical messengers (cytokines) that regulate the intensity of the immune response. These cytokines may include interleukin-1, interleukin-6, and tumor necrosis factor (TNF), which are potent inflammatory agents that worsen joint inflammation and contribute to disease progression.

Five of the most widely available drugs in this category—etanercept (Enbrel), infliximab (Remicade), adalimumab (Humira), golimumab (Simponi), and certolizumab (Cimzia)—work by blocking the action of TNF, and they work relatively fast. More recent additions to the category of biologics target other cytokines involved in RA.

Oftentimes, biological response modifiers are given in combination with methotrexate to help provide both immediate and longer-term relief (see Box 3-6, "Methotrexate/biologic combo helps save large joints").

Etanercept (Enbrel)

In a 2014 study, the combination of etanercept and methotrexate resulted in greater reductions in disease activity and greater rates of RA remission within two weeks compared to methotrexate use alone, although no significant differences in the number of tender or swollen joints were reported after one year.

Infliximab (Remicade)

Of those taking infliximab and methotrexate in one study, 60 percent of those with RA showed improvement when given a high dosage, and 50 percent improved with a lower dosage. Use of the drug combo even seemed to limit disease progression in those who had RA for 10 years or more.

Adalimumab (Humira)

This drug can be taken alone or in combination with DMARDs, and is given by injection once every two weeks. A 2014 study found that 70 percent of patients given adalimumab plus methotrexate had achieved low RA disease activity after 78 weeks, compared to 54 percent of patients given methotrexate alone. Adalimumab is approved for treating active RA as well as early-stage RA (defined as being within three years of initial diagnosis).

Golimumab (Simponi)

A 2014 study found that adding subcutaneous golimumab to traditional DMARD therapy improved treatment responses and remission rates among more than 3,000 RA patients treated with non-biologic DMARDs.

Certolizumab (Cimzia)

This drug has a different chemical structure than other TNF-blockers, which allows it to remain active in the body for longer periods of time and may allow it to go directly to the inflamed joint. A small study (*Annals of the Rheumatic Diseases*, June 2015) found that certolizumab reduced synovitis and osteitis (bone inflammation) among 36 RA patients over 16 weeks. Earlier research found that certolizumab plus methotrexate produced improvements in symptoms and function over five years.

Overall there is no convincing data that one TNF-blocker is better than another. They are generally well tolerated, but, like all medications, they carry risks of side effects (see "Biological Response Modifiers/Side Effects," page 39).

Anakinra (Kineret)

Unlike the other biological response modifiers described here, anakinra acts by blocking the action of interleukin-1, an important mediator produced in areas of inflammation. By inhibiting interleukin-1, the drug helps block the release of proteolytic enzymes that would otherwise degrade the cartilage. It is less effective than the TNF antagonists, so it is not used commonly in the treatment of RA.

Tocilizumab (Actemra)

Tocilizumab blocks the inflammatory cytokine interleukin-6. Offered as an infusion or subcutaneous injection, the drug is generally well tolerated, but it may cause elevated liver enzymes, increased levels of LDL ("bad") cholesterol, high blood pressure, and gastrointestinal perforations. The most common side effects reported in clinical trials of tocilizumab were upper respiratory tract infections, headache, nasal inflammation, high blood pressure, and increased liver enzymes, according to the FDA.

JAK inhibitors

Biologic response modifiers are given by injection or infusion, but new drugs known as janus kinase (JAK) inhibitors offer RA relief in pill form. Kinases serve as gatekeepers of the immune system that regulate the degree of an inflammatory response produced.

Tofacitinib

The first of these drugs, tofacitinib (Xeljanz), gained FDA approval in 2012 for people with moderate-to-severe RA who do not respond adequately to methotrexate or cannot tolerate it. (Other JAK inhibitors are in development.) A 2014 study found that tofacitinib was superior to methotrexate in reducing RA symptoms and inhibiting the progression of joint damage among 958 patients with no prior use of methotrexate.

A major selling point of tofacitinib is that it's a pill, making it more attractive for RA patients who need biologic medications but aren't fond of injections or infusions. However, the drug's twice-a-day dosing schedule may be problematic for people who have difficulty adhering to a medication regimen. Dosing of the other biologic drugs for RA ranges from weekly to as infrequently as every four to six months. Like other biologic DMARDs, tofacitinib may increase the risk of serious infections, tuberculosis, and cancers such as lymphoma. Clinical trial data suggest that the rate of shingles may be higher with tofacitinib compared to the other biologic drugs. Tofacitinib may cause low blood counts and increases in cholesterol and liver enzymes, so, as with other biologic drugs, you must undergo periodic monitoring with blood tests while on treatment.

Cell blockers

Instead of blocking specific proteins produced by immune cells, some RA drugs block activation of key immune cells (T cells or T lymphocytes).

Abatacept (Orencia)

One of these drugs—abatacept (Orencia)—is in a class of compounds called co-stimulator blockers, which block one of the two molecules needed to activate a T cell. A 2014 study found that some patients treated for 12 months with abatacept (with or without methotrexate) achieved remission from their RA without medications at 18 months. The drug is administered via intravenous infusion or subcutaneous injection, both of which work equally well.

Rituximab (Rituxan)

Rituxan, administered via intravenous infusion in combination with methotrexate, is recommended to treat patients with moderate-to-severe RA who have not improved with TNF antagonists. Rituxan selectively targets immune cells known as CD20-positive B cells, which are believed to play a role in RA inflammation. Research suggests that 1) rituximab remains well tolerated and has a favorable safety profile after 9½ years, and 2) rituximab plus methotrexate can slow joint damage in early RA compared to methotrexate alone, even among patients with moderate and high levels of disease activity.

Biological response modifiers/side effects

Because biological response modifiers suppress the immune system, those who take them are more prone to infections, especially of the upper respiratory tract. In fact, use of TNF inhibitors has been linked to increased risk of tuberculosis. A 2014 study found that rates of bacterial infections were similar among the biologic drugs, but were higher with infliximab. However, other research suggests that the risk of serious infection posed by TNF inhibitors is no greater than that associated with non-biologic DMARDs.

Similarly, the evidence is mixed as to whether use of TNF inhibitors increases the risk of herpes zoster, or shingles. Guidelines from the American College of Rheumatology and other experts recommend that patients be vaccinated against herpes zoster before starting therapy with traditional DMARDs or biologic drugs (but patients already taking biologic drugs should not receive the vaccine). However, in a study presented at the American College of Rheumatology's 2014 Annual Scientific Meeting, researchers reported that among about 300 patients treated with biologic therapy for RA and other inflammatory conditions, a strategy of withholding one dose of a biologic drug and replacing it with the vaccine was safe and did not increase the incidence of shingles over six weeks.

Your doctor must help you weigh the risks and benefits of using these drugs. They should not be taken by people who have an active infection, and they need to be used with caution by those who have a history of recurrent infection or who are generally more susceptible to infection.

As with the findings related to the infection risks associated with TNF inhibitors, the literature is mixed on whether the use of these drugs increases the risk of certain cancers that are already known to be elevated in people with RA. An analysis of 71 clinical trials involving 23,456 patients found an increased risk of non-melanoma skin cancer but no greater risk of other malignancies associated with adalimumab use after nearly 12 years. And, an analysis of data involving 114,291 patients found no increased risk of melanoma associated with TNF inhibitors (American College of Rheumatology Scientific Meeting, November 2014). Regardless, the labels for TNF inhibitors contain warnings about increased cancer risk associated with use of the drugs.

A review of the evidence

One meta-analysis examined the adverse effects associated with the TNF inhibitors, abatacept, anakinra, rituximab, and tocilizumab. The analysis included more than 200 studies encompassing nearly 62,000 patients who were followed for a median of six to 13 months. According to the study, compared to people who received a placebo, those given a biologic drug:

▶ Will probably experience more side effects or drop out of a study due to side effects than those taking a placebo.

▶ Are more likely to develop tuberculosis. Twenty out of 10,000 people taking a biologic drug developed tuberculosis, compared to four out of 10,000 for placebo patients.

▶ Will probably not experience more serious side effects, serious infections, cancer, or heart failure.

The analysis found that, compared to placebo patients, those given infliximab were significantly more likely to experience a side effect (777 out of 1,000 versus 724 out of 1,000) and drop out of a study due to side effects (181 out of 1,000 versus 98 out of 1,000).

Finding the right drug combination

The right combination of NSAIDs, corticosteroids, DMARDs, or biological response modifiers varies greatly, depending upon your age, level of disease, overall disability, and general medical condition.

Arriving at the optimal mix that controls symptoms, prevents progressive joint damage, and reduces harmful side effects is largely trial and error, and may require a year or more to refine. Individual response varies widely, so it is essential that you work with your rheumatologist in choosing and customizing your treatment. Some research has found that in people who don't respond to methotrexate alone, adding two additional DMARDs to the drug is just as effective as adding a TNF inhibitor. Other research has found that this triple-DMARD strategy is more effective than methotrexate alone for newly diagnosed RA, but a high percentage of patients treated with this approach eventually discontinue it.

Tapering therapy

Researchers are exploring strategies aimed at gradually reducing the dosage, lengthening the interval between doses, or halting therapy altogether in patients who achieve remission from RA using biologic therapy, in an effort to minimize the side effects and costs (see Box 3-7, "Tapering, stopping RA treatment may be feasible").

In a study published Nov. 6, 2014, in the *New England Journal of Medicine*, RA patients who achieved remission after a year of treatment with 50 mg of etanercept plus methotrexate were then given half the combination dose, methotrexate alone, or a placebo for 39 weeks. Those who stayed in remission on the half-dosing regimen then had all treatment withdrawn for another 26 weeks. At the end of this period, 44 percent of the combination-therapy group were still in remission, compared to 29 percent of the methotrexate group, and 23 percent of the placebo group, the study found. The study authors suggest that after achieving remission or low RA disease activity with early, aggressive treatment, "a reduction in or withdrawal of biologic therapy may be reasonable in some patients, particularly those who have sustained remission."

Most drug therapies for knee osteoarthritis (OA) pain are more effective than placebo, but injections of hyaluronic acid (HA) appear to be the most efficacious, according to a 2015 meta-analysis. Researchers reviewed 137 studies (comprising more than 33,000 participants with knee OA) that compared two or more of the following: acetaminophen, celecoxib, diclofenac, ibuprofen, naproxen, oral placebo, and injections of HA, corticosteroids or a placebo. All of the treatments, except acetaminophen, produced clinically significant improvements in knee pain, with HA the most effective, followed by steroid injections. The researchers suggested that the beneficial effects of the injections may be due, at least in part, to the method of drug delivery, because placebo injections also were effective, even more so than oral NSAIDs.

Annals of Internal Medicine, Jan. 6, 2015

Viscosupplements/cushioning fluid

When a knee lacks sufficient lubricating fluid (synovial fluid), due to mild-to-moderate arthritis or age, doctors may inject a thick viscous substance (hyaluronic acid) into the joint space to provide temporary lubrication and pain relief. This process, known as viscosupplementation, is largely used for OA.

Though the U.S. Food and Drug Administration (FDA) has officially approved the use of viscosupplements only for the relief of knee OA, it's quite common for physicians to recommend these injections for ankle or elbow pain.

Six months or longer of relief

Viscosupplements may provide effective and long-lasting pain relief (up to six months) in 90 to 95 percent of those with mild-to-moderate knee OA. For those with more severe OA, the injections are significantly less effective.

The injections are generally well tolerated. The most common side effects are post-treatment inflammation or swelling at the injection site, though this is usually manageable with ice and anti-inflammatory medications. Your doctor may recommend that you stay off your feet for the first day or two after an injection, and to ice your knees each of those days.

Though it may take two to three months before you get maximum benefit from the injections, patients claim they also get immediate pain relief, possibly because the viscosupplement coats the pain receptors in the knee.

However, studies have produced conflicting findings about the efficacy of viscosupplements. One study concluded that viscosupplementation offers little benefit, while increasing the risk of serious adverse events. Conversely, a 2015 study comparing oral and injectable treatments for knee arthritis found that viscosupplementation appeared to provide the greatest benefit (see Box 3-8, "Injections helpful for knee OA"). Other research revealed that the injections significantly delayed the need for total knee replacement among 14,000 patients.

A few concerns

Since the hyaluronic acid in most viscosupplements is derived from chicken combs, those with a severe allergy to chicken or eggs may want to avoid them, although there are no reports that support such concerns. These injections should not be used in tandem with other injections, such as those of cortisone or lidocaine.

Finally, cost is a factor. A single course of treatment with a viscosupplement costs at least $500. Many insurance providers cover the cost of treatment, although some require that you try other conservative therapies first. Still, see if your private insurance carrier will reimburse you.

PRP: The healing power of blood

Your blood's own natural healing capabilities form the basis of platelet-rich plasma (PRP) injections. In these treatments, a sample of blood is removed, and the platelets and growth factors are separated from the red blood cells and injected in a solution back into the site of injury.

PRP is used most often to treat tendon injuries. However, some small studies have suggested some benefit of treating arthritis in the knee or other joints with PRP. Since PRP uses your own blood, the treatment is generally safe, although most patients have soreness immediately after the injection, sometimes lasting for the first week or two.

Prolotherapy/tightening problem tissues

If loose ligaments and tendons cause pain, then the advocates of prolotherapy believe that tightening up these lax tissues can help solve the problem. In this procedure, the problem area is given a series of injections of dextrose solution over time. The intent is to cause localized inflammation and scarring (sometimes called sclerotherapy or regenerative injection therapy) in the tissue, in order to tighten it and trigger new tissue growth and increased blood supply. One study involving 90 people with knee OA found that the treatment provided improvements in pain, function, and stiffness for up to a year. However, more research is necessary before prolotherapy can be considered as a replacement for more clinically proven medical and surgical treatment of arthritis.

Other drug therapies
Topical treatments
Lidocaine patch (Lidoderm)
The lidocaine patch is a prescription-only patch that contains a local anesthetic and is now widely used by arthritis patients for flare-ups

of back pain, and for pain around large joints. Because the patch is relatively large (5 x 6 inches), it is not suitable for smaller joints, such as the finger or wrist. The patch may remain in place for up to 12 hours in any 24-hour period. However, it is expensive, with a pack of 30 costing nearly $300 in some cases.

Fentanyl patch (Duragesic): powerful, but use with caution

These prescription-only transdermal patches contain fentanyl, a very potent narcotic, and are intended as a long-term way to help manage severe, chronic pain. The slow-release patches (eight to 12 hours) are designed to be changed every three days.

Misuse of the patches poses a risk of overdose. Risks are particularly high if you replace the patches more frequently than the instructions indicate, use the patches when you drink alcohol, or have an increase in body temperature or are exposed to heat from sources like heating pads, electric blankets, heat lamps, saunas, hot tubs, or heated water beds. Signs of overdose include breathing difficulties, extreme fatigue, and feelings of faintness or dizziness.

Celadrin/cetylated fatty acids

Some research suggests that a topical cream that contains cetylated fatty acids (CFAs) rapidly eases the pain of OA and improves range of motion and mobility. Though researchers are unsure exactly how CFAs work, they believe they reduce chronic inflammation by reducing the release of the key immune system messengers interleukin-1 and leukotriene B4.

Drugs used for other purposes

Researchers also are studying drugs approved to treat other diseases for use in arthritis, including drugs normally used to treat osteoporosis. Some evidence suggests that the bisphosphonate drug risedronate may protect bone in patients with knee OA, while another bisphosphonate, zoledronic acid, may prevent bony erosions in RA.

Some research suggests that cholesterol-lowering statin drugs may reduce the risk of developing RA, while other studies have suggested that RA patients who took statins had significantly lower disease activity, lower levels of the inflammatory marker C-reactive protein, and fewer swollen joints, compared to those who weren't taking the medications.

Gene therapy: Getting joint cells to make their own drugs

Though doctors can give drugs, such as the biological response modifier anakinra, to block the action of interleukin-1 and shut down the release of cartilage-destroying enzymes, researchers may soon teach joint cells to make their own protective drugs. Investigators have inserted genes into the joint cells of animals that make a harmless protein that parks itself on the outer surface of key immune system cells, thus preventing them from "switching on" and releasing their destructive enzymes. Research on gene therapy for arthritis continues.

New biologics

Some other biologics for RA that are under study include:

▶ Drugs targeting other cytokines: Drugs like tocilizumab block the action of interleukin-6, and scientists are developing new medications—such as clazakizumab, sarilumab, and sirukumab—that also affect this same biologic pathway in differing ways. Research suggests that experimental drugs that block other inflammatory cytokines, including inter-leukin-17 and interleukin-20, also may help treat RA.

▶ B-cell depletors: While Rituxan is already approved for moderate-to-severe rheumatoid arthritis, other B-cell-depleting drugs remain under study. Like Rituxan, the new drugs target B-cells, which are cells of the immune system that are believed to play a role in causing inflammation in rheumatoid arthritis. These drugs bind to the surface of B-cells, effectively killing them off.

▶ Small molecule inhibitors against cytoplasmic kinases: Tofacitinib is the first JAK inhibitor already approved for RA treatment. Several others are under investigation in the JAK family, as well as agents against other kinases.

▶ Biosimilars: Researchers are developing medications that are similar to biologic response modifiers in terms of quality, safety, and efficacy, but have small, structural differences. Interest in these biosimilar drugs has grown because of expectations that these compounds will be more cost-effective than the original versions. But, because of the subtle differences between the biosimilars and their originators, some experts have raised concerns about the efficacy and safety of these new drugs. However, research presented in 2014 found that a biosimilar of etanercept was comparable to the original drug in terms of efficacy and safety, as was a biosimilar of infliximab. Research into the development of biosimilar drugs continues.

INTRODUCTION TO JOINT SURGERY

If medications, physical therapy, exercise, and weight control aren't enough to manage the pain, stiffness, and functional declines caused by arthritis, it's time to think about surgery. But first, consider how significantly your arthritis is affecting your quality of life, and how much benefit you'll gain from surgery. Get all the facts about what the surgery entails, and what you can expect afterward in terms of rehabilitation and recovery time.

From arthroscopy to total joint replacement, surgeons can employ a variety of techniques to ease joint pain and improve function. Which procedure is right for you depends on the type and severity of arthritis you have, the joint affected, your age and overall health, and the amount of functional improvement you require (see Box 4-1, "Signs it may be time for joint surgery," and Box 4-2, "Questions to ask before deciding on surgery," on the following page).

Today's less-invasive surgeries allow for shorter hospital stays (although some surgeries are now outpatient procedures) and faster recovery times. Technological advances in designs, materials, and surgical techniques have improved the success of joint replacements, and surgeons are following new protocols to reduce the cardiovascular risks after joint-replacement surgery.

Joint surgery for the knee and hip
Synovectomy
Synovectomy, the surgical removal of the entire lining (synovium) of a damaged knee joint, is occasionally recommended for those in the early stages of RA. The lining is removed via open surgery or arthroscopically, eliminating the source of excess fluid production and inflammation that leads to swelling and pain. However, synovectomy is often not a cure since the lining may grow back within a few months, with the problem returning.

Arthroscopy
Getting rid of arthritis pain by having debris washed out of your knee joint or having its lining scraped (debridement) are common options.

More than 330,000 total hip replacements are performed in the U.S. each year.

BOX 4-1

Signs it may be time for joint surgery

- Insufficient pain relief with medications, weight loss or physical therapy

- Taking part in fewer daily activities due to joint pain

- Difficulty going up or down the stairs, getting up out of a chair, or off the toilet due to joint pain

- Difficulty walking more than a few blocks because of joint pain

Questions to ask before deciding on surgery

Though joint surgery is an increasingly common procedure, it remains a major decision requiring a lot of thought. Here are some questions to ask yourself and your doctor before deciding on surgery:

- Can I bear the pain I'm experiencing now? Does it significantly limit what I can do?

- What other treatments could I have instead of surgery?

- What are the risks of surgery? What are the risks if I don't have surgery?

- How much pain will there be during the surgery? What about afterward?

- Can the surgery be done on an outpatient basis? If not, how long can I expect to stay in the hospital?

- How long is the recovery process? Am I prepared to work through the recovery stages, including physical therapy and exercise, as required?

- How much will surgery help my condition? Realistically, how much improvement can I expect?

- What limits will there be on my activities (driving, bending, climbing stairs) and for how long?

- Does my insurance fully cover the cost of surgery and recovery? If I have out-of-pocket expenses, can I afford them?

- Will I be able to take the time off needed to recover from surgery?

- What medications will I need after surgery, and how long will I need to take them?

- Can I talk to several previous patients of my age and condition who have recently gone through the surgery?

But when it comes to pain relief, these procedures may not provide long-lasting benefits unless there are loose bone fragments or torn cartilage. Arthroscopy is best for fixing mechanical problems in your knee, such as repairing torn cartilage or removing bone chips. It's not a solution for arthritis pain (see Box 4-3, "Arthroscopic surgery no help for mild knee OA"), and some research suggests it's no better than physical therapy or medications for people with moderate-to-severe knee arthritis.

Joint replacement

The primary reason to consider joint replacement (arthroplasty) for arthritis is pain that disrupts your daily life and does not respond to other treatments. Of all the surgical options, only joint replacement is viewed by doctors as a long-term cure. The surgery is being performed today in record numbers, and is projected to increase exponentially in the next two decades, outpacing the number of surgeons who can perform these operations. The procedure resurfaces the damaged joint, which afterward depends upon remaining muscles and ligaments for support.

How long do joint implants last?

When first used in the 1970s, joint implants lasted about 10 years. Today, with better surgical techniques, improved prosthetic designs, and stronger materials, most joint implants can be expected to last 20 years or more. And researchers continue to develop better designs that aim to give you near-normal range of motion and function for the rest of your active life.

The plastic now used in artificial hips, knees, and ankles is 20 times more durable than the material used just a few years ago. In some of the latest hip systems, the ball at the end of the femur stem and the liner of the pelvic cup are made of ceramic—not the ceramic of brittle pottery, but rather an extremely hard, durable form of aluminum: aluminum oxide.

Friction is the main enemy of implant life, because particles produced by friction can work their way between bone and implant, gradually eroding the bone and loosening the artificial joint. How the replacement joint is affixed to the surrounding bone also may determine how long the implant lasts.

Knee replacement

When to consider knee replacement

For patients with severe knee arthritis, the pain needs to be bad enough to make the risk of surgery justifiable. Such pain often makes it difficult to walk more than a few blocks, take part in normal daily activities, or sleep through the night without waking due to the pain. As the degeneration worsens, it can also damage the underlying bone and lead to deformities such as knock-knees or bowlegs. One study found that nearly a third of patients undergoing total knee replacement experienced a rapid worsening of their knee OA and symptoms in the two years leading up to their surgery.

Unicompartmental or partial knee replacement

Unicompartmental replacement is similar to total knee replacement in that the worn surfaces within your knee are replaced by metal and plastic parts. However, rather than realign and resurface both the medial (inside) and lateral (outside) compartments of the knee joint as in total knee replacement, the unicompartmental, or partial, knee replacement resurfaces and replaces only the medial or lateral compartment of the knee. In both surgeries, the end of the femur and the top of the tibia are replaced.

This partial approach is considered mainly in younger patients and in older patients to shorten their recovery period. It makes sense only when your arthritis is confined to one compartment of your knee.

Compared to those receiving a total knee replacement, partial knee replacement patients may recover faster. For older patients, it helps with knee stability, since you keep all of your ligaments intact. On the downside, it tends to wear out faster than a total knee replacement—in as little as 10 years, compared to 20 with a total knee implant. However, if a unicompartmental replacement fails, it can be converted to a total knee replacement with a second operation.

Total knee replacement

Total knee replacement is the only procedure in which you remove everything that is, or could become, diseased—the

---

TOTAL KNEE REPLACEMENT

A total knee replacement is composed of several parts:

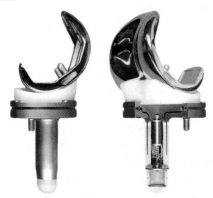

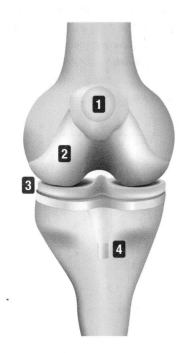

1 A plastic patellar button that gets cemented to the underside of the kneecap.

2 An upper (femoral) component made of metal alloy that fits into the end of your thigh bone (femur).

3 A hard plastic piece, an insert that snaps into the lower metal component and sits between your two metal-clad bones, acting as a new artificial cartilage.

4 A lower (tibial) component, a T-shaped piece of metal that fits into your lower leg bone.

cartilage, the linings, and the ends of the bones (see Box 4-4, "Total knee replacement"). Research suggests that total knee replacement can ease pain, and improve physical and social functioning, balance, and vitality in older adults. Some studies have found that replacing a knee or hip may reduce the risk of cardiovascular complications, probably because the surgery improves a person's capability for physical activity, thus improving cardiovascular health. Other research has found that most patients who undergo total knee replacement are able to return to work, even heavy labor.

Minimally invasive total knee replacement

An effective operation, traditional total knee replacement entails cutting through muscles and tendons around the knee, a long and sometimes painful recovery, and a significant scar. In minimally invasive total knee replacement, the surgeon does not cut the quadriceps muscle but instead spreads apart the muscle fibers and uses smaller instruments to make cuts to the bone similar to those in traditional total knee replacement.

A smaller incision and less cutting of tendons and muscles allows for faster recovery. At four to six weeks, the average range of motion for minimally invasive surgery patients is 15 to 20 percent greater than for those getting traditional total knee replacement.

On the downside, working through a smaller incision is surgically challenging, making it more difficult to achieve precise cutting angles and optimal anatomic alignment between bone and implant. Some studies have shown a higher rate of complications with minimally invasive versus traditional knee replacement.

It's all about alignment

The long-term success of your new knee requires that it be precisely aligned with your femur and tibia in order to allow optimal transfer of force across it—the key to reducing the risk of premature wear and loosening.

The large incision of traditional surgery makes such measurements relatively straightforward, but achieving such precision gets more difficult as the incision gets smaller. As such, getting good alignment with a minimally invasive approach is challenging because the surgeon has a harder time ensuring perfect anatomic alignment, especially if there is previous scarring or anatomic deformity. For this reason, if you've had previous knee operations, or are severely bow-legged or knock-kneed, a traditional approach is frequently recommended.

Computers and customization

At some larger medical centers, surgeons are using computer-aided navigational tools to help achieve more precise alignment when doing minimally invasive knee replacement as well as certain types of traditional knee replacement. However, the benefits of computer-navigated versus conventional total knee replacement remain unproven.

Surgeons align the knee-replacement components with the help of anatomical landmarks in the patient's knee at the time of surgery. However, not all knees are the same, and getting the joint aligned properly can be difficult in patients with deformities and other knee abnormalities. So, researchers are studying customized knee replacements with instrumentation tailored to the individual patient's knee anatomy.

Similarly, some knee replacement prostheses are too wide for patients with small frames, such as petite women, causing the implant to extend over the bone. This overhang has been associated with pain after knee replacement surgery. Anatomic differences between men and women have led to the development of narrower, gender-specific knee implants. The hope is that these custom implants will reduce surgical margin of error, offer improved function, and reduce the risk of implant failure requiring revision surgery—however, research has yet to show any major difference in clinical and functional outcomes between these prostheses and traditional knee replacement systems.

Rehabilitation and recovery

Evidence in recent years shows that people having minimally invasive surgery can recover in about half the time as those with traditional knee replacement, without any apparent reduced risk of long-term success. This means being able to walk without a cane or get out of bed or a chair unassisted in perhaps three to four weeks, instead of needing six to eight weeks.

Improvements in surgical techniques and recovery protocols

BOX 4-5

Getting the most from a total knee replacement

- **Prevent infection:** Discuss with your surgeon the need to take antibiotics before dental work or any invasive procedure that breaks the skin and adds to infection risk.

- **Reduce impact:** Avoid activities (such as running, singles tennis, and racquetball) that put repetitive stress on your knee and accelerate wear.

- **Lose weight:** Every extra pound puts at least three pounds of additional force across your knee.

- **Exercise your leg muscles:** Walk, swim, or lift weights to strengthen the muscles and ligaments around your knee, but avoid strenuous loading, such as leg presses that may involve very heavy weights.

have led some experts to recommend shorter hospital stays or even outpatient procedures for joint replacement patients. The theory is that cutting the typical three- to four-day hospital stay down to one or two (or none at all) may reduce the risk of post-operative complications, such as infections.

You can take steps to get the most out of your knee replacement (see Box 4-5, "Getting the most from a total knee replacement"). Your conditioning going into your knee replacement may affect the speed and quality of your recovery. For instance, research suggests that taking part in physical therapy—or "prehabilitation"—before joint replacement may help improve recovery and reduce the need for care at a rehab center or skilled nursing facility after surgery (see Box 4-6, "Prehab may reduce need for post-operative care after joint replacement"). Other evidence suggests that the presence of co-morbid conditions, such as obesity, may increase the risk of post-operative complications or the need for repeat joint surgery. For instance, a study presented in 2014 found that people with metabolic syndrome—a constellation of risk factors including abdominal obesity, high blood pressure, high triglycerides, low HDL cholesterol, and insulin resistance—were more than twice as likely as those without the syndrome to experience a complication in the hospital and/or within one year of surgery. Other evidence suggests that if you smoke, you're more likely to experience complications from total joint replacement surgery.

Medications after surgery

Medications and physical therapy also may help speed your recovery. One study found that taking celecoxib around the time of the operation led to a more rapid and less painful recovery from total knee replacement, while another found that physical therapy on the day of surgery shortened hospital stays significantly among those undergoing knee or hip replacements. Conversely, another study found that people taking opioid pain relievers—such as hydrocodone (Vicodin, Lortab) and oxycodone (OxyContin)—before surgery had longer hospital stays, lower function, and less mobility in the replaced knee, and more pain, stiffness and complications two to seven years after surgery.

Fear of pain and re-injury can inhibit recovery after knee

surgery, often resulting in avoidance of physical activity and the development of decreased muscle strength, limited range of motion, weakness in the cardiovascular system, and weight gain. A study presented in 2014 found that weight gain after knee or hip replacement was associated with lower scores on post-operative assessments of pain, functioning, and activity, while patients who lost weight scored higher on these evaluations.

Bilateral knee replacement

If both of your knees are arthritic and painful, you might need to have them both replaced. The question is whether to have them replaced simultaneously (a procedure known as bilateral knee replacement) or in separate, staged operations. Bilateral knee replacement is attractive because it means one operation, one anesthesia, and one recovery period. Once you've recovered, you have two new joints that, ideally, will allow you to resume your normal activities. On average, patients undergoing bilateral surgery need four to six months before returning to normal activities.

Having your knees replaced separately means one surgery and then another one no sooner than three to six months later. With each surgery, a typical patient requires three months to return to normal activities, meaning six months' total recovery time associated with two surgeries. Data suggest that bilateral and unilateral patients do equally well in the long term, and, generally, the life expectancy of the implant is the same (about 15 to 25 years). With either approach, you can resume sports (e.g., golfing, tennis, walking, swimming), but your doctor may advise against high-impact activities, such as competitive basketball, running, and downhill skiing.

Some risks

The downside is that the initial recovery period and rehabilitation after bilateral surgery can be much more difficult because you don't have a "good leg" to work with. Many bilateral patients first must go to a rehabilitation center before they're able to return home.

The major potential drawback is the risk associated with the surgery itself. More surgery means more bleeding and an increased need for blood transfusions. As such, your doctor may have you donate blood beforehand to be given as a transfusion during surgery. Bilateral surgery also has been associated with a slightly higher risk of cardiac events (such as heart attack) and deep vein thrombosis (DVT), a blood clot that forms in the leg veins. With increased DVT risk comes a slightly greater risk that the clot will travel to the lungs, resulting in a potentially deadly pulmonary embolism.

Due to these potential complications, bilateral surgery is not for anyone with a history of DVT, pulmonary embolism, or cardiovascular complications, such as heart disease, heart attack, stroke, or revascularization (bypass surgery or angioplasty with stenting). And, it may not be appropriate for some morbidly obese patients. Generally, ideal candidates for bilateral surgery are healthy adults under age 75.

Preventing cardiac complications after joint replacement

Experts are working to find the best ways to reduce clot formation and identify people at greater risk of cardiac problems after joint replacement. In fact, a 2014 study found that deaths from heart attack, stroke, venous blood clots, and other causes declined by nearly two-thirds between 1989 and 2007.

The FDA has approved several drugs to prevent blood clots and related complications after joint replacement surgery: apixaban (Eliquis), enoxaparin (Lovenox), fondaparinux (Arixtra), heparin, rivaroxaban (Xarelto), and warfarin (Coumadin). Some evidence suggests that aspirin and cholesterol-lowering statin drugs also may help prevent deep vein thrombosis and pulmonary embolism after surgery.

Blood-thinning medications can be risky because they're associated with excessive bleeding. An alternative is a mechanical compression device that wraps around the leg and pumps it to promote blood flow, but these cumbersome devices, available only in hospitals, prevent walking. However, a smaller, battery-operated device can be used outside the hospital.

The American Academy of Orthopaedic Surgeons recommends that all patients undergoing joint replacement surgery receive anticoagulant therapy and/or mechanical compression devices, although evidence is insufficient to advocate any particular preventive strategy or duration of treatment. The experts also recommend that patients consider having their surgery under regional anesthesia—which causes less blood loss and, potentially, fewer complications than general anesthesia—and that they get up and walk as soon as safely possible after the operation.

Older adults and people with a history of cardiac problems—including coronary artery disease, heart attack, heart failure, irregular heartbeats, and heart-valve disease—are at increased risk of developing cardiac complications after knee and hip replacement surgery. As described earlier, bilateral surgery (having both joints replaced during the same operation) may increase the risk of cardiovascular complications, as may revision surgery (removing an existing prosthetic joint and replacing it with a new one).

Some research suggests that cardiovascular and other post-surgical complications also may be more likely among people with uncontrolled diabetes, and that better blood-sugar control before, during, and after surgery may result in fewer complications.

Hip replacement
Goal of hip implants

More than 300,000 total hip replacements are performed in the U.S. each year. Research suggests that total hip replacement not only eases pain, but also may help patients resume or begin a more active lifestyle after surgery. Another study found that, compared to people with hip osteoarthritis who did not have a total hip replacement, those who underwent the surgery had lower rates of death, heart failure, depression, and diabetes, although their risk of cardiovascular disease was increased in the year after the operation.

The goal of total hip replacement is to replace the worn surfaces of the ball-and-socket joint. Typically, the upper head of the femur is replaced by a metal ball mounted on a metal stem that is placed firmly into the canal of the thighbone. The worn hip socket is replaced with a metal cup that, in turn, is fitted with a plastic insert. It is against this plastic insert that the metal ball rotates as you move. Ideally, this insert is made of a material that

BOX 4-7

TOTAL HIP REPLACEMENT

A total hip replacement is composed of several parts:

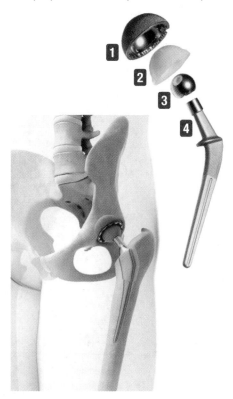

1 A socket component, which is usually made of strong metal.

2 A polyethylene or ceramic liner, which allows the artificial hip joint to move smoothly.

3 A metal or ceramic ball that replaces the ball (femoral head) at the top of the thighbone.

4 A metal stem that fits inside a hollowed-out channel in the thighbone.

has a low frictional resistance and wear rate against the metal ball (see Box 4-7, "Total hip replacement").

Why hip implants wear out

Unfortunately, the liner used in most hip inserts, though made of high-density plastic (polyethylene), still degrades over time. Not only does the plastic liner wear, but it also sheds tiny particles. These particles find their way to the spot where the implant is anchored into the bone, and can cause irritation. The body reacts to this irritation by trying to remove the particles and, in the process (known as osteolysis), it removes a little bit of bone as well, slowly loosening the implant. Over time, this erosion creates the need to surgically revise the implant. These revision surgeries are more difficult than the original, and their success is more limited.

Although this wear and tear is most often the cause of prosthetic joint complications, studies have found that dislocation and infection are other common reasons why the implants fail. Other evidence suggests that hip implants may be more likely to fail in women than in men, and that patients with rheumatoid arthritis may be at greater risk of dislocation after hip replacement compared to their osteoarthritis counterparts.

Metal-on-metal concerns

The pursuit of a longer-lasting hip prosthesis prompted renewed interest in devices employing a cobalt-chrome head bearing against a smooth metal pelvic cup. Proponents say these metal-on-metal implants improve the durability of hip replacements, cut down on debris, provide better range of motion, and allow for larger femoral heads, which may reduce the risk of dislocation. But research has found a higher failure rate among some metal-on-metal designs, as metal particles from the implants can trigger adverse reactions in the hips of some patients. The FDA reports that in rare cases, metallic ions entering the bloodstream may have caused illness elsewhere. In general, metal-on-metal implants are not recommended for women of childbearing age, and for patients who have kidney problems, are on high-dose corticosteroid therapy, have a known allergy/sensitivity to metals, or have a suppressed immune system.

In 2013, the FDA issued a safety communication, recommending that orthopaedic surgeons consider metal-on-metal hip implants only after determining that the risk-benefit profile outweighs that of using another type of hip implant system.

The FDA also issued the following recommendations for patients who already have metal-on-metal hips:

▶ If you have no symptoms and your orthopaedic surgeon believes your implant is functioning appropriately, routinely follow up with the surgeon every one to two years. (Note: The FDA does not recommend that asymptomatic patients undergo routine imaging studies or tests for metal ions in the blood.)

▶ If you develop new or worsening problems such as pain, swelling, numbness, noise (popping, grinding, clicking, or squeaking of your hip), and/or a change in your walking ability, contact your orthopaedic surgeon immediately.

▶ If you experience changes in your general health, including new or worsening symptoms outside your hip (e.g. chest pain, shortness of breath, numbness, fatigue, or changes in urination habits), let your physician know you have a metal-on-metal hip implant.

Despite these concerns, the American Academy of Orthopaedic Surgeons notes the following about metal-on-metal hip implants: "Although the exact prevalence of adverse reactions to metal debris is not known, current experience leads us to consider the adverse outcomes to be relatively low or equal (with some designs) to other types of hip implants. Thus, for many patients, currently available information supports a favorable risk-benefit ratio."

Minimally invasive hip replacement

While traditional total hip replacement requires an incision that is, on average, 10 to 12 inches long, the incision for a minimally invasive (aka "mini-hip") replacement is approximately three to four inches in length. This is often enough to enable the surgeon to see the ends of your femur and the cup, or acetabular, part of your pelvis. However, in larger, obese patients, the incision may need to be lengthened in order to allow the surgeon to see around the additional fat tissue.

Mini-incision vs. mini-invasive

Just because a hip replacement is performed through a smaller incision doesn't necessarily make it less invasive. Some surgeons offer a "mini-incision" approach, but they end up essentially doing traditional surgery through a smaller opening.

To be truly minimally invasive, a surgeon must not only make a smaller incision, but must also reduce the number of underlying muscles and tendons cut. Rather than sever (and eventually suture back) many of these muscles and tendons that connect to the head of the femur, in a minimally invasive approach, the surgeon cuts away only a few of these tissues, and works around or between the remaining muscle bundles to position the implant.

The frontal approach

In a newer approach to total hip replacement, called minimally invasive direct anterior surgery, the surgeon places the hip prosthesis through a four- to six-inch incision at the front of the hip instead of at the side or the back (posterior). The procedure spares the muscles and tendons around the hip, and it doesn't require the array of precautions that patients must take after conventional hip replacement.

Proponents say the anterior approach has several advantages over traditional surgery, including less pain and a need for less pain medicine, shorter hospital stays, a quicker recovery, and fewer postoperative restrictions. And, unlike conventional hip replacement, the anterior approach can be done with the guidance of intraoperative fluoroscopy, which provides real-time X-ray images of the hip.

Experience counts

Working through a small incision poses additional challenges for the surgeon, since he or she must be able to confidently navigate using a somewhat restricted field of view, yet still precisely position the parts of the hip implant.

Such confidence in tight quarters comes largely through practice. So if you're having mini-hip surgery, or any joint replacement, you're better off in the hands of a surgeon who does a high volume of these procedures. One study found that the need for revision surgery to correct a problem with the initial surgery was 22 percent higher among surgeons who performed fewer than 12 hip replacements a year compared to those who performed more annually. Have the procedure at a center that specializes in hip replacement surgery, and ask your surgeon how many procedures he or she has performed and what is his or her revision rate.

Recovery rates vary

With a mini-hip procedure, you can generally expect to recover faster than if you've had traditional hip replacement, because it's the healing and reconditioning of the cut and reattached tendons and muscles that require the most time. The standard is six weeks for a mini-hip and 12 weeks for a traditional replacement, although those recovery times are growing shorter (see Box 4-8, "Two-week return to driving for most hip-replacement patients").

Using a minimally invasive approach will increase your chance of a faster recovery, but it doesn't guarantee it. Your recovery depends upon your overall health and fitness prior to surgery, as well as your motivation for sticking with rehab afterward. The less fit you are before surgery, the longer your recovery will take, no matter what approach is used.

Hip resurfacing

Unlike total hip replacement, which removes the head and neck of the femur and replaces them with a metal ball and stem, hip resurfacing keeps the neck intact and resurfaces and reshapes the head, covering it with a metal cap. Both procedures require a cup to be placed in the hip socket (acetabulum).

On the positive side

Surgeons who perform the procedure claim it allows for greater range of motion than total hip replacement and preserves the normal hip mechanics, and they may recommend it for younger, more active patients who still have healthy bone stock. Research suggests that the rate of complications from hip resurfacing is lowest in men under age 55. Proponents note that the large head of the hip resurfacing system makes it more difficult than a traditional hip prosthesis to dislocate, which means that

Two-week return to driving for most hip-replacement patients

Improvements in surgical techniques, pain management, and rehabilitation protocols have enabled patients undergoing total hip replacement to return to driving as soon as two weeks after surgery, according to a recent study. Before surgery, 38 people who had their right hip replaced between 2013 and 2014 underwent tests to measure how quickly they could react to a stimulus and apply the brakes. They repeated these tests at two, four, and six weeks after the surgery, and were allowed to resume driving when their post-operative braking time was equal to or less than their pre-operative time. Of the 38 patients, 33 (87 percent) reached their pre-operative braking time within two weeks, while the rest achieved it at four weeks.

American Academy of Orthopaedic Surgeons Annual Meeting, March 2015

resurfacing patients may not have to follow all the precautions—such as avoiding bending forward more than 90 degrees or crossing their legs—that their hip-replacement counterparts do in the weeks after surgery. And, should the resurfacing fail, the prosthesis can easily be converted to a total hip replacement.

On the negative side

As with metal-on-metal total hip replacements, wearing of the metal-on-metal hip resurfacing system may produce metallic ions that causes synovitis (inflammation of the hip joint lining), and may eventually lead to loosening and failure of the device. Also, one study found that metal debris from hip resurfacing caused adverse tissue reactions known as pseudotumors (non-cancerous lesions in the tissue surrounding the resurfacing components) in 28 percent of 143 hip resurfacings. Although most of these growths were asymptomatic, seven patients required revision surgery because of a symptomatic pseudo-tumor, the researchers reported.

What concerns U.S. surgeons most is that with resurfacing, there is a risk of fracturing the femoral neck, which is left intact and is usually the weakest part of the natural hip joint. Such a risk doesn't exist with total hip replacement because the neck is replaced with metal. Approximately one to two percent of those who have hip resurfacing will have such a fracture, usually within four months of surgery. This may occur because the remaining bone is not healthy enough, so older patients and people with osteoporosis may not be suitable candidates for resurfacing. Or the femoral neck may fracture because the cap and cup are not fitted precisely enough to allow normal transfer of forces across the joint. One study found that the risk of revision for hip resurfacing at eight years was significantly greater than that for conventional total hip replacement, except for men under age 55 with osteoarthritis who required a larger femoral component size.

Joint surgery for shoulder arthritis

About 53,000 people have shoulder replacement surgery each year, and one study concluded that people who undergo the procedure can expect significantly fewer complications, shorter hospital stays, and less cost than their counterparts who have knee or hip replacement. Still, the success of shoulder replacement (and all orthopaedic surgeries, in general) depends greatly on the experience of the surgeon and the surgical center. A study published Nov. 4, 2014, in *Arthritis Care & Research* found that patients who underwent the operation at hospitals that performed more than 15 total shoulder replacements a year had shorter hospital stays, were less likely to suffer complications such as post-surgical fracture, and were less likely to need revision surgery, compared to patients who had the surgery at lower-volume centers.

In total shoulder replacement, a metal ball attached to a metal stem driven into the humerus (upper arm bone) bears against a plastic cup fitted inside the glenoid socket of the shoulder (see Box 4-9, Shoulder replacement"). In some cases, such as when the ball of the humerus is severely fractured but the socket is normal, the surgeon may perform a partial (hemi) replacement and replace only the ball. Complication rates are similar between the two procedures, one study suggests.

Historically, shoulder replacement was mostly an option for older, inactive patients with advanced osteoarthritis and an intact rotator cuff. But surgeons today can offer a wider range of options matched to the age, disease state, and activity level of each patient.

Shoulder resurfacing

In shoulder resurfacing, or partial shoulder replacement, instead of removing the entire end of the upper arm bone (humerus) and replacing it with a metallic ball and stem, the natural bone is left in place and the ball is reshaped and fitted with a metallic cap. In addition, the natural indentation in the glenoid cavity, in which the humerus sits to create the shoulder joint, is not replaced with a hard plastic polyethylene cup. Rather, the surgeon creates a cup made from material taken from elsewhere in your body (such as a piece of fibrous tissue from your outer thigh).

The use of such a natural-tissue cup reduces the risk of implant failure due to friction particles. Such extended longevity of a shoulder implant is particularly important in the resurfacing approach, since the technique is largely reserved for younger, more active patients.

BOX 4-9

SHOULDER REPLACEMENT

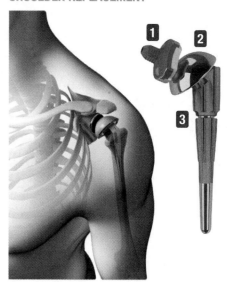

A shoulder replacement is similar to a hip replacement, and consists of:

1 Plastic cup/glenoid component.

2 Implant ball.

3 Humeral stem.

Reverse shoulder system

Other advances, such as the reverse shoulder system, are helping older patients retain greater shoulder mobility with less pain. With this system, the normal positioning of the shoulder components is transposed, with the metal ball (glenosphere) and stem fitted into the glenoid cavity and the hard plastic cup on top of a stem fitted into the top of the humerus.

This reverse system is designed mainly for patients with severe arthritis who can't raise their arms due to severe rotator cuff tears. Its design allows the intact and still strong muscles in other parts of the shoulder, such as the deltoid muscle, to take over the work of the damaged rotator cuff and help hold the implant together more tightly than the injured shoulder can. The result is a more stable shoulder that is less likely to dislocate.

Joint surgery for arthritic wrists
Wrist fusion

This surgery eliminates motion between parts that are often the cause of ongoing pain.

For active arthritis patients who have only one or two bones rubbing together in the wrist, partial wrist fusion may be appropriate. In this procedure, the surgeon fuses together the problem bones using wires or metal plates and fills intervening spaces with bone graft to help the bones grow together. Newer advances are improving fusion rates by allowing multiple screws to be anchored to each bone. Compared to total wrist fusion, partial fusion can preserve more motion in the wrist.

In another operation, proximal row carpectomy, the row of bones closer to your forearm is removed, and your new wrist or bend point moves closer to the fingers. This procedure is usually for older arthritis patients who don't require high use of the wrist.

If partial fusion or proximal row carpectomy doesn't provide adequate pain relief for your arthritis, the surgeon can do a full or total fusion of the wrist. Once fused, you can't bend the wrist, but are able to rotate it 180 degrees, turning your palm up or down.

Wrist replacement

Joint replacement in the wrist can be an option for some patients with severe arthritis who do not need to use their wrist for heavy daily use. Unlike fusion surgery, wrist replacement may help maintain or recover wrist movement, and it may help improve the ability to perform daily activities.

Wrist replacement surgery can be done as an outpatient procedure. Patients will wear a cast for several weeks, followed by a protective splint for another six to eight weeks. Patients must do exercises to restore movement and increase strength and endurance in the wrist. According to the American Academy of Orthopaedic Surgeons, wrist replacement can improve motion to about 50 percent of normal, and a typical wrist replacement can be expected to last 10 to 15 years with careful use.

Joint surgery for foot and ankle arthritis
Try other options first

Our feet and ankles are anatomic jigsaw puzzles containing more than 25 percent of the bones in our bodies. When injury or disease causes even one piece to shift slightly out of place, stress can begin to wear at any of the 30 joints in the foot, and arthritis may follow (see Box 4-10, "Foot and ankle bones").

Fortunately, such arthritis can usually be detected early, and in most cases managed with a combination of medication and orthotics (shoe inserts), braces, and splints to relieve pain and restore proper alignment. However, if pain persists, surgery may be necessary.

Debridement and fusion

In the very early stages of ankle arthritis, the surgeon can go in with a scope and clean out (debride) the joint, removing any bony outgrowths or other debris.

In the later stages of foot and ankle arthritis, bone fusion remains the standard surgical procedure. The goal is to eliminate the motion causing the pain. In fusion, the surgeon removes the cartilage between the offending bones, then uses stainless steel rods, screws, or plates to join them as one. Total ankle replacement, however, is becoming a good option for certain patients with ankle arthritis.

BOX 4-10

FOOT AND ANKLE BONES

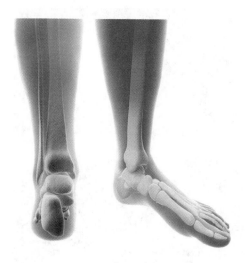

The feet and ankles contain more than 25 percent of the bones in the body. The foot alone includes approximately 30 joints, all of which may be susceptible to arthritis.

BOX 4-11

ANKLE REPLACEMENT

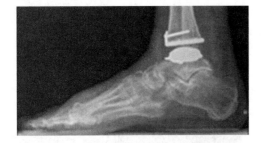

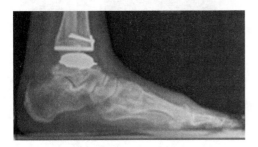

Ankle replacement surgery replaces the lower end of the tibia (shin bone) and the top of the foot bone (talus) with metal components. A mobile bearing made of polyethylene fits between the metal parts, to act as a shock absorber and reduce friction.

Ankle replacement surgery

The ideal patients to receive a total ankle replacement are older, relatively inactive people with debilitating end-stage arthritis who are not diabetic and who do not smoke.

One study found that ankle replacement provides greater improvement in physical functioning and quality of life compared to ankle fusion surgery. Unlike ankle fusion, total ankle replacement preserves motion and, in doing so, may better protect joints adjacent to the ankle from arthritic changes that may occur years after ankle fusion (see Box 4-11, "Ankle replacement"). With advances in designs, including patient-specific instrumentation used to better customize the operation for the individual patient, most of today's total ankle replacements can be expected to last at least 10 years. But, as with any orthopaedic surgery, the experience and skill of the surgeon, as well as individual patient characteristics and rehabilitation, play key roles in determining the success of total ankle replacement.

Other surgical developments
Knuckle replacement

Knuckle implants may help patients in the early stages of rheumatoid arthritis, younger patients with post-traumatic arthritis, or older patients with osteoarthritis who put high, repetitive stress on the joints. New, two-piece designs—made from either metal and plastic, or pyrolytic carbon—are engineered to last longer and restore a greater level of function than traditional silicon implants.

With either of the new designs, a candidate must have plenty of healthy bone on both sides of the knuckle, as well as enough healthy soft tissue to provide stability.

For the thumb

Neither of these newer implant designs is used to replace a diseased thumb joint, since that joint is inherently less stable. Typical surgery to treat thumb-base arthritis requires the surgeon to remove the bone at the base of the thumb, and either temporarily pin the joint or place a piece of tendon in the space.

Some people who need more strength and stability in the

finger or thumb may require surgical fusion of the bones in the problem joint. In some cases, the surgeon may recommend a combination of replacement in some finger joints and fusion in others.

Spinal disc replacement

Select patients with lower back pain have an alternative to spinal fusion in the form of an artificial lumbar disc (see Box 4-12, "Lumbar disc replacement"). Some research suggests that lumbar disc replacement is comparable to or slightly better than spinal fusion at easing pain and improving function (see Box 4-13, "Long-term results favorable for lumbar disc replacement").

Lumbar disc replacement is not for everyone. Candidates should have a diagnosis of serious degenerative disc disease in only one disc region in the lumbar spine and have had at least six months of prior conservative treatment. Patients also must be in overall good health, with no signs of osteoporosis or infection.

Disc replacement in the neck

A number of artificial discs are approved to treat problems associated with degenerative disc disease in the neck. While relieving neck and arm pain, artificial cervical discs also are designed to maintain neck motion and, as a result, avoid the loss of mobility and the degeneration of adjacent discs that can occur with spinal fusion. A study published online Feb. 28, 2015, in *The Spine Journal* found no significant differences between cervical disc replacement and cervical spinal fusion in terms of disability or complication rates among 137 patients in the two years after surgery.

The discs are intended to relieve symptoms requiring surgical treatment at only one cervical level. Patients should be aware that cervical disc replacement, like other spinal surgeries, is recommended only after conservative treatment options have been exhausted.

Cartilage repair

Joint replacements can work wonders if you have significant cartilage degeneration from arthritis. But if the damage is

BOX 4-12

LUMBAR DISC REPLACEMENT

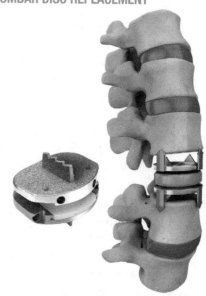

Artificial discs typically have two metal plates, one of which is attached to the vertebra above, while the other is attached to the vertebra below. Between the metal parts is a compressible plastic "spacer" that allows for movement and shock absorption.

NEW FINDING BOX 4-13

Long-term results favorable for lumbar disc replacement

In a small study, most patients who received a lumbar total disc replacement continued to experience improvements in pain and disability for more than a decade. For an average of about 12 years, Chinese researchers followed 35 patients who received a lumbar disc replacement. They reported that 28 of the patients had a successful outcome, according to the U.S. Food and Drug Administration (FDA) criterion of greater than 25 percent improvement in measures of pain and disability. Two patients required a follow-up surgery: one because of degenerative changes in the spine segment adjacent to the disc implant, the other due to a pedicle fracture. However, "The results of our long-term follow-up indicate that, with strict indication, [lumbar disc replacement] is a safe and effective procedure as an alternative to lumbar fusion," the researchers concluded.

European Spine Journal, online April 21, 2015

BOX 4-14

Cartilage repair: A youthful pursuit

In all the cartilage repair procedures in use or under study, treatment is aimed primarily at young patients (under age 40) with traumatic arthritis due to injury. This is because the procedures require a large amount of healthy bone and cartilage for extraction and reuse. Unfortunately, for most people in their 60s with advanced arthritis, their joints are badly worn, little healthy tissue remains, and their overall health is not robust enough to support cartilage regrowth.

In general, the new cartilage is not as durable as the body's natural hyaline cartilage. Patients undergoing any cartilage repair remain on crutches for several weeks and use continuous passive motion therapy—in which the joint is gently moved by a machine—for several hours a day.

limited to a small area, you may not need such a major operation. Enter cartilage regeneration (see Box 4-14, "Cartilage repair: A youthful pursuit"). Several procedures can stimulate the growth of new cartilage-like repair tissue, relieve pain, and improve joint function, although questions remain about the durability of this new tissue.

Microfracture regrowth

The most common cartilage-repair procedure, microfracture, entails clearing tissue debris from the joint and creating tiny holes (microfractures) in the subchondral bone underlying the damaged cartilage. Bone marrow then seeps out through these holes, carrying mesenchymal stem cells that mix with the blood clot that develops. This process results in the formation of a repair cartilage called "fibrocartilage," which is not as durable as the original cartilage.

Creating a paste of cartilage cells

In a procedure known as autologous chondrocyte implantation (ACI), a surgeon uses arthroscopic surgery to harvest cartilage cells, which are then sent to a laboratory, cultured by the millions for four to six weeks, and are sent back to the surgeon as a paste. In a second operation, the surgeon implants the cells back into the joint and removes a piece of periosteum (the membrane that covers the bone's outer surface) to seal the cells in place. A related procedure, matrix-induced autologous chondrocyte implantation, or the MACI procedure, involves harvesting cells, growing them onto a backing membrane called a matrix, and transplanting the matrix to the bone.

Cartilage plugs

Another technique, osteochondral autografting (mosaicplasty), entails the removal of one or more cylindrical plugs of cartilage and bone from a healthy, non-weight-bearing part of the joint. (If a cartilage defect is too large, a tissue graft taken from a cadaver donor may be used.) The plugs are then transplanted into a damaged area in the knee, ankle, or shoulder, like fixing potholes in the cartilage. In a similar procedure, osteochondral autograft transfer system, or OATS, the plugs are typically larger, and thus only one or two are needed to repair the cartilage damage.

Cartilage scaffolds

Researchers are trying to find a better way to mend the small cartilage tears suffered by competitive athletes, using sponge-like scaffolds made of collagen. The 3D scaffolds provide a lattice-work to hold the new cartilage cells in place as the joint heals while being used. Tissue engineers have developed a scaffolding procedure that encourages a torn meniscus to repair itself. Otherwise, this cartilage, which acts as the knee's shock absorber, will not heal. In an analysis of 13 studies, published in the May 2015 issue of *Arthroscopy*, researchers concluded that implanting collagen scaffolds to treat meniscus defects "provides satisfactory clinical and structural outcomes in most cases."

Cartilage gel

Researchers have grown cartilage cells in a gel, outside the body, and then used the gel to patch similar tiny fissures in the cartilage. In this approach, the gel is implanted arthroscopically and, once in place, begins to slowly break down, giving the seeded cartilage cells enough time to integrate with the remaining joint cartilage.

Other investigations involve an injectable synthetic cartilage hydrogel that mimics the body's own chondrocytes to help repair damaged cartilage. Scientists say the gel is pliant but incredibly durable, and won't degenerate even when deformed more than 1,000 percent. Results of a pilot study showed that in 15 patients given a hydrogel scaffolding and adhesive implant during microfracture surgery, new cartilage had filled an average of 86 percent of the defects in their knees after six months. In three patients treated only with microfracture, an average of 64 percent of the defective tissue was replaced. Patients given the hydrogel implant also reported a greater decrease in knee pain during the follow-up period.

Enter gene therapy

Scientists are testing gene therapy as a way to direct stem cells to grow into functional cartilage. In a new procedure, engineers genetically altered stem cells placed on a synthetic cartilage scaffolding to produce growth factor proteins necessary to form cartilage. In 2014, the researchers reported that the new technique may pave the way for the development of bioactive implants that grow at the site of tissue repair, circumventing the need for tissue generation outside the body.

SUPPLEMENTS AND OTHER LESS TRADITIONAL OPTIONS

If your arthritis still affects your daily life despite a combination of medications, diet, exercise, and other conventional therapies, it's natural to seek solutions in the form of complementary and alternative medicine. From herbal and dietary supplements to acupuncture and spinal manipulation, to mind/body techniques, a wide range of complementary and alternative treatments has been touted to ease arthritis pain and improve function.

Some of these treatments are supported by clinical research, while others are backed mostly by limited anecdotal evidence. Nevertheless, experts typically consider these therapies as a complement, not a substitute, for traditional medicine. And, because many of these less conventional options have not been rigorously studied and validated through clinical testing, approach them with a certain amount of caution.

General advice on supplements
Lack of quality control

Because dietary and herbal supplements, unlike drugs, are not regulated by the Food and Drug Administration (FDA), there is no standardization of just what may be in the bottle, and no proof of their safety or effectiveness. For example, in 2015, the New York Attorney General's Office ordered four national retailers to remove certain store-brand herbal supplements from their shelves after tests showed that many products contained no traces of the herbs indicated on the labeling. The products often contained fillers such as houseplants and powdered rice. Similarly, in a 2013 study, Canadian researchers found that nearly six out of 10 herbal products contained plant species not listed on the label, and only two of the 12 manufacturers submitted products without fillers, contaminants, or cheaper herbs that substituted for the active ingredient. Other studies have found traces of heavy metals, insecticides, and pesticides in some botanicals.

FDA regulations do not permit sellers of dietary supplements to claim that their products can treat, prevent, or cure specific

If you opt to take supplements that claim to ease arthritis, let your doctor know so he or she can alert you to possible interactions with medications you're already taking, as well as side effects.

diseases. Yet, a U.S. Government Accountability Office (GAO) report found that manufacturers of a number of dietary supplements commonly used by older adults made deceptive or questionable marketing claims about their products.

To get some semblance of quality control, it's probably best to go with large national manufacturers of supplements, since they have an investment in maintaining a good reputation. Another safety strategy is to look for products with labels that bear the symbol of independent testing organizations, such as ConsumerLab.com or U.S. Pharmacopeia, which measure supplements for quality, strength, and purity.

Read labels carefully

The FDA does require supplements to have labels that are easy to read and understand and, like food, to list ingredients in order of decreasing quantity. By reading labels carefully you can compare brands for strength, dosage and price. You also want to be wary of exaggerated claims, especially supplements that promise immediate results, outright cures, or even the ability to treat many types of arthritis. Arthritis is not just one disease, and any supplement that claims to treat multiple forms of it should be suspect and probably avoided.

Let your doctor know what you're taking

Be up front about every treatment you are taking, including over-the-counter drugs, vitamins, diet pills, nutritional supplements, or any other alternative treatments. Just because something is "natural" doesn't mean it's safe or without side effects. Doctors need to know the full list so they can alert you to possible interactions with medications you're already taking, as well as side effects, such as increased bleeding risk. Bleeding is of particular concern because many people with arthritis take aspirin or other nonsteroidal anti-inflammatory drugs (NSAIDs), which slow the rate at which blood clots. The use of herbal supplements, some of which have anti-clotting effects, can slow this rate further. Those already taking prescription blood thinners, such as warfarin (Coumadin), are advised to avoid the use of supplements altogether.

Supplements: Specifics
Glucosamine

Glucosamine sulfate is among the most widely used arthritis supplements, particularly for osteoarthritis (OA), and is usually taken in combination with chondroitin. Glucosamine is a normal component of cartilage produced in your body, and is believed to play a role in stimulating your cartilage cells to make new collagen and proteoglycans.

Although glucosamine, which is made from seashells and coxcombs, is rapidly absorbed in the gastrointestinal tract when you swallow a tablet, only a small percentage of the glucosamine gets carried by the blood to the target joint.

Who may benefit

Results of the largest study of glucosamine and chondroitin ever conducted—the $14 million NIH-sponsored Glucosamine/Chondroitin Arthritis Intervention Trial (GAIT)—found that people with mild-to-moderate OA who took the supplements showed no more relief than if using placebo. However, those with more advanced disease (moderate-to-severe arthritis) did report significant pain relief (25 percent better than placebo) when using the supplement combo.

Later phases of GAIT found that none of the study treatments produced clinically significant improvements in pain or function compared to placebo, but "glucosamine and chondroitin showed beneficial but not significant trends."

Many rheumatologists suggest that if you have moderate-to-severe OA pain, there is little harm in trying glucosamine and chondroitin with your doctor's approval, and some patients have reported improvements while taking the supplements (see Box 5-1, "Studies support benefits of glucosamine and chondroitin"). Based on previous study findings, the suggested dosage is 1,500 milligrams (mg) of glucosamine per day. For optimal absorption, take 500 mg three times a day. It can take up to three months before you start to see the benefits, but most physicians suggest you stop taking it if you see no difference after 10 weeks of use.

NEW FINDING   BOX 5-1

Studies support benefits of glucosamine and chondroitin

Two recent clinical trials suggest that glucosamine and chondroitin may ease pain and inhibit cartilage loss in knee osteoarthritis (OA). In one study, 606 people with moderate-to-severe knee OA pain were assigned to receive glucosamine and chondroitin or the prescription pain reliever celecoxib every day for six months. At the end of the study, both treatment groups had experienced about a 50 percent reduction in pain and comparable improvements in joint stiffness and function. In the second study, 605 people with chronic knee pain and evidence of knee OA received glucosamine, chondroitin, both supplements, or a placebo, and were followed for two years. The researchers found that use of the supplement combination, but not the individual supplements or placebo, resulted in a significant reduction in joint space narrowing, a sign of cartilage deterioration and advancing OA. All of the treatment groups reported reduced knee pain, but there were no differences between the supplement groups and those who received a placebo.

Annals of the Rheumatic Diseases, January 2015, May 2015

BOX 5-2

Supplement dos and don'ts

- **Think big:** Buy from national companies that have a major investment in maintaining their reputation.

- **Look for a symbol:** Look for labels that carry the symbols of independent testing organizations, which help ensure consistent contents.

- **Tell all:** To help reduce bleeding risk and other complications, tell your doctor about every supplement, diet pill, nutrient, and herbal treatment you're taking.

- **One at a time:** Try only one supplement at a time; you can better gauge its effect this way. Stop after three months if there has been no impact.

- **Don't believe the hype:** Don't select supplements based on testimonials or claims. You want facts.

- **Don't fall for one-size-fits-all:** Avoid supplements that claim to be effective against osteoarthritis, rheumatoid arthritis, gout, and other forms of arthritis. These are unique diseases requiring unique treatments.

- **Don't stop your meds:** Supplements are just that, and not substitutes for traditional medicine. Keep taking your prescribed medications.

- **Don't assume natural is safe:** All supplements have the potential to interact with your body and the drugs you're taking, creating cross-reactions such as increased bleeding risk.

Possible side effects

Though most people have no side effects from glucosamine, a few may experience gastrointestinal discomfort, drowsiness, skin reactions, or headache. If you're allergic to shellfish, you need to be careful with the source of the glucosamine, since some brands are derived from lobster shells. If you're diabetic, you also need to be careful, since glucosamine is an amino sugar and, theoretically, could make it harder to manage your blood sugar. Glucosamine can also slightly increase your risk of bleeding, since it makes the platelets in your blood a bit less likely to clot. Those already on a blood-thinning medication, such as warfarin (Coumadin), should probably avoid taking glucosamine altogether.

Herbal supplements

Herbal medicine is an age-old practice with modern consequences. For thousands of years, people have been using parts of plants or their extracts to heal what ails them (for tips on supplement use, see Box 5-2, "Supplement dos and don'ts."). Some 25 percent of current prescription drugs are derived from plants, and the list of non-prescription herbal remedies is even longer. Some of them claim to relieve arthritis pain—however, high-quality evidence supporting the use of herbal supplements for OA pain is generally lacking or unconvincing.

One unproven herbal arthritis remedy is pine bark extract (pycnogenol). Although some earlier studies suggested the supplement may significantly reduce OA symptoms, a large review of studies concluded that the evidence supporting the use of pycnogenol for any medical condition is insufficient to make any conclusions about its efficacy and safety.

Some research suggests that herbal Ayurvedic medicine (popular in India) is equally as effective as glucosamine or celecoxib (Celebrex) at improving knee OA pain and physical function, with fewer adverse effects. And, another study found that Ayurvedic therapy was comparable to methotrexate in easing symptoms and improving function in patients with rheumatoid arthritis (RA).

Consider medication interactions

If an herbal treatment can help control your pain, you may also be able to reduce your dependence on nonsteroidal anti-inflammatory drugs (NSAIDs), and lower your risk of side effects. But herbal medicines also pose side effects of their own. If an herb is able to have an effect on your arthritis, it also may have an impact on other systems in your body.

Herbal supplements can reduce the effectiveness of disease-modifying antirheumatic drugs (DMARDs) like methotrexate. People already on blood thinners or anticoagulants need to be aware of supplements that claim to be anti-inflammatory, since they may be similar to aspirin and could add to your bleeding risk.

In several reports, researchers have reviewed the evidence from dozens of clinical trials on herbal supplements for arthritis. Here are a few summaries of what they found:

Gamma linolenic acid (GLA)

GLA is a type of omega-6 fatty acid found in evening primrose oil, black currant seed oil, and borage seed oil, which is believed to help reduce the joint pain, stiffness, and swelling associated with RA. A 2014 study found that use of GLA, with or without fish oil, resulted in reductions in RA disease activity and the use of RA medications. An earlier analysis concluded that GLA reduced pain intensity and improved disability, without a significantly increased risk of side effects. However, GLA is an anticoagulant that could increase the risk of bleeding if taken with blood-thinning medications or NSAIDs.

Thunder god vine

Although not widely available in the U.S., extracts of the roots of the medicinal vine Tripterygium wilfordii Hook (thunder god vine), used in Traditional Chinese Medicine, have been shown to confer some benefits in people with autoimmune disorders, and inflammatory conditions such as RA. In a 2014 study, thunder god vine was about as effective as methotrexate for reducing RA disease activity, and a combination of the two treatments was even better. However, the doses of methotrexate used in the study were lower than what is typically used for RA, and the study was not long enough to assess whether thunder god vine prevents joint damage. Note that thunder god vine has a wide range of side effects (mostly gastrointestinal), and can be toxic if not carefully extracted from the skinned root. Other parts of the plant are poisonous and potentially lethal, according to the National Center for Complementary and Integrative Health.

Avocado-soybean unsaponifiables (ASU)

A 2014 study found that among 399 people with hip OA, ASU (a mixture of avocado and soybean oils) appeared to reduce progressive deteriorating joint space width, a measure of advancing arthritis. Other studies have shown significant pain relief and improved mobility, as well as a reduction in the need for NSAIDs, in people with hip or knee OA.

Devil's claw

Limited evidence supports the use of devil's claw, the root of a traditional herbal plant from Africa. Since stomach acid may neutralize the effects of harpagoside (the active ingredient in devil's claw), the herb should be taken between meals. Possible side effects include lowered blood pressure, as well as interference with blood-thinning, cardiac, and diabetes medications.

SAM-e

A synthetic form of a natural byproduct of the amino acid methionine, S-adenosyl-methionine (SAM-e, pronounced "Sammy") is widely used in Europe, where it is sold as a drug. Some earlier U.S. clinical studies suggest that it may work as well as NSAIDs in relieving OA pain and improving mobility. Overall, though, a review of the medical literature found that the evidence to support the use of SAM-e is lacking, and additional studies are needed.

Vitamin therapy

Antioxidant vitamins

Vitamin C, vitamin E, and beta-carotene are inflammation-fighting antioxidants, so the belief is that they may be helpful against arthritis. Vitamin C also helps in the formation and maintenance of collagen and other connective tissue. However, though normal daily amounts of vitamin C (90 mg a day for men and 75 mg a day for women) and vitamin E (15 mg a day) are necessary, taking even more of the vitamins may be counterproductive in the fight against OA. In a 2014 study involving more than 3,000 people, those who had the highest blood levels of vitamin C and E were significantly more likely to develop knee OA over a 30-month follow-up period. Earlier, a major Australian study found that vitamin E and vitamin C were no more effective than a placebo at reducing joint wear or cartilage loss due to arthritis.

Vitamin C may have a role in reducing the risk of another inflammatory arthritis: gout. One study found that men with higher intakes of vitamin C through food and supplements had a reduced risk of gout, while another found that vitamin C supplementation significantly reduced levels of uric acid, which can accumulate and form crystals that cause gout pain. However, another study found that vitamin C had no clinically significant effect on reducing uric acid levels in 40 patients with gout.

Clearly, more research is needed to make a convincing case in support of antioxidant vitamin therapy for arthritis. Note that vitamins can become toxic in megadoses, and taking too much vitamin E can have an anticoagulant effect, promoting bleeding.

Vitamin D

Getting enough vitamin D is essential if you are trying to maintain or build strength and endurance in an osteoarthritic knee. In fact, one investigation found that nearly half of patients undergoing orthopaedic surgery have a vitamin D deficiency. Similarly, a 2015 study found that more than three-quarters of RA patients had low vitamin D, and this deficiency was associated with worse disease activity and quality of life.

Some evidence suggests that vitamin D deficiency not only increases pain but also is associated with loss of knee cartilage (see Box 5-3, "Higher vitamin D levels linked to lower OA pain"). However, results of a randomized, controlled trial published in 2013 found that vitamin D provided no benefit for patients with knee OA.

Since the elderly are less efficient at producing vitamin D from sunlight and absorbing it from food, they may require a vitamin D supplement. Most experts—including the National Osteoporosis Foundation and the International Osteoporosis Foundation—now recommend getting 800 to 1,000 international

Higher vitamin D levels linked to lower OA pain

Obese people with knee osteoarthritis (OA) may function better if they get ample levels of vitamin D, recent research suggests. The study included 256 middle-aged and older adults who were queried about their knee OA pain and underwent tests of their vitamin D levels and their lower extremity function. Compared to those with vitamin D deficiency or insufficiency, the participants with adequate vitamin D levels reported significantly less knee OA pain, regardless of their weight. And in obese patients, those with adequate vitamin D levels could walk, balance, and rise from sitting to standing better than obese participants with insufficient levels.

Clinical Journal of Pain, January 2015

Real acupuncture no better than fake treatment for knee pain

Adding to earlier evidence, a recent study found that acupuncture doesn't improve knee pain any more than fake ("sham") acupuncture. In the study, nearly 300 adults with chronic knee pain received needle acupuncture, laser acupuncture (hitting acupuncture spots with a low-intensity laser beam), sham laser acupuncture, or no treatment at all. After receiving 20-minute sessions up to twice a week for three months, participants receiving needle, laser, or sham acupuncture all experienced similar reductions in knee pain while walking, compared to the non-treatment group. Neither needle acupuncture nor laser acupuncture provided significantly greater pain relief than sham laser acupuncture.

Journal of the American Medical Association, Oct. 1, 2014

units (IUs) of vitamin D a day. The U.S. Institute of Medicine recommends 600 IUs of vitamin D per day for people under age 70, and 800 IUs for those over 70. A cup of milk has about 100 IUs, three ounces of cooked salmon has 794, and one cup of vitamin D-fortified orange juice has about 100.

Fish oil

Fish oil contains antioxidants (omega-3 fatty acids) that some people think can help prevent arthritis. Some studies seem to suggest fish oils can help with OA, and that omega-3 fatty acids might decrease the pain and swelling of RA. Research suggests that consuming omega-3 fatty acids—found in fatty, oily fish like salmon, mackerel, herring, and tuna—can improve RA symptoms and potentially reduce the risk of developing RA. In one study, researchers studied the use of fish oil supplements, combined with triple DMARD therapy, in patients with early-onset RA. They found that failure of triple DMARD therapy was lower and rates of RA remission were greater in patients given high-dose fish oil compared to those given a low, clinically ineffective dose.

Some evidence suggests that cod liver oil may be beneficial to OA and RA patients. In one study, researchers found that the supplement reduced NSAID use among 97 RA patients by 30 percent over a nine-month period, and patients experienced no worsening of their disease related to decreased NSAID use.

How much is enough?

Omega-3 fatty acids are the main ingredient of cod liver oil. The Food and Nutrition Board of the U.S. National Academy of Sciences has established a minimum daily requirement for omega-3: 1.1 grams a day for adult women, and 1.6 grams a day for adult men. When taking any fish oil supplements, read the label to determine how much omega-3 is in each gel cap, as indicated by the amounts of EPA (eicosapentaenoic acid) and DHA (docosahexaenoic acid).

Acupuncture

Acupuncture, a 2,000-year-old Eastern practice that involves the insertion of thin needles into the body at strategic points, has become one of the most accepted alternative therapies. Scientists believe that the twirling of the needles along known acupuncture points (meridians) stimulates nearby nerves, causing a variety of effects, including release of endorphins, the natural painkilling hormones that block pain messages from reaching the brain. The number of hospitals offering acupuncture has grown; however, its effectiveness seems to be more established for some types of pain than others.

Good for knee osteoarthritis?

A 2014 study found that six weeks of thrice-weekly acupuncture treatments using moxibustion (in which a Chinese herb is burned in a small device placed near acupuncture sites) was effective at reducing pain and improving function in patients with knee OA. However, other studies have found no difference between genuine and fake ("sham") acupuncture for knee OA (see Box 5-4, "Real acupuncture no better than fake treatment for knee pain").

It may be best to combine acupuncture with traditional medical therapy. In one study, researchers found that standard medical care plus 15 sessions of acupuncture reduced pain and improved quality of life.

May help with lower back pain

Compared to standard medical treatment, acupuncture may be better for chronic lower back pain (see Box 5-5, "Acupuncture provides short-term help for chronic back pain"). In one study, researchers found that among 187 people with low back pain, those given standard or Hegu acupuncture (using needling points specifically in the hand) reported better scores on assessments of disability and pain compared to those given usual care. Other research suggests that genuine and sham acupuncture may be similarly beneficial for low back pain.

No replacement for standard care

Most clinicians suggest acupuncture should be used in combination with standard care, not as a replacement (see Box 5-6, "What to do if you're considering acupuncture"). People with bleeding disorders and those who take blood thinners

Spinal manipulation may ease back-related leg pain

Recent research suggests that spinal manipulative therapy may provide short-term improvements in pain and function from back-related leg pain, such as sciatica. In the study, 192 people age 21 and older, with back-related leg pain lasting at least four weeks, were randomized to receive 12 weeks of home exercise and advice about simple pain-management techniques, or exercise/advice combined with spinal manipulation. The participants were evaluated 12 weeks after the treatment ended and again at one year. Compared to the participants who received home exercise/advice alone, those who received spinal manipulation plus home exercise/advice gained more pain relief, were less likely to have low back pain and disability, and were less likely to use pain medications at 12 weeks, but the benefits were not sustained at one year. However, the spinal-manipulation group reported better satisfaction with their care at both time points.

Annals of Internal Medicine, Sept. 16, 2014

such as warfarin (Coumadin) should avoid acupuncture, as should those who are HIV-positive, or who have hepatitis B infections, skin infections, valvular heart disease, pacemakers, or cardiac arrhythmias.

Spinal manipulation

Approximately 40 percent of patients with acute lower back pain initially see a chiropractor, not their physician, when the pain occurs. There is some evidence that manipulation or chiropractic adjustments can provide relief (see Box 5-7, "Spinal manipulation may ease back-related leg pain"). One randomized trial found that patients receiving a form of spinal manipulation known as osteopathic manual therapy (OMT) used less pain medication, were significantly more likely to report moderate or substantial improvements in low back pain, and were more likely to be satisfied with their back care compared to those given fake OMT.

Although spinal manipulation is generally safe, people with osteoporosis should avoid more vigorous high-velocity, low-amplitude manipulation. Concerns also have arisen from reports of more vigorous cervical (neck) manipulation causing vascular injury, stroke, and death. Overall, the risk of these injuries is low, and some instances have occurred in patients who had not undergone an X-ray of the cervical vertebrae that might have uncovered reasons not to do manipulation.

Heat therapy

Applying heat to a painful joint can help increase blood flow, provide local pain relief, ease muscle spasms, and improve flexibility. Also, heating joints and muscles with hot packs or towels, or by taking a warm bath or shower before exercising, may help you exercise more easily.

Many patients believe mud baths help relieve arthritis pain, and though no specific studies have been done to show this, it makes sense that a warm mud bath would be a good way to reduce stress, promote relaxation, and improve circulation.

Heat treatments are appropriate when inflammation is not evident. If inflammation is present, ice may be more effective.

Cold therapy

Using cold to numb the nerves around a sore joint is another way to relieve inflammation, ease muscle spasms, and reduce pain. Cold therapy can involve cold packs, ice massage, soaking in cold water, or over-the-counter sprays and ointments that cool the skin and joints. Cold is commonly used in the acute states of RA, since lowering the temperature of inflamed joints to 86 degrees Fahrenheit (30 degrees Celsius) or lower helps reduce the activity of cartilage-destroying enzymes common to RA.

Hydrotherapy

This is an ancient practice, also known as spa therapy or balneotherapy, which uses mineral baths to soothe pain. Mineral baths—like mud or heat therapy—seem a logical way to improve circulation and reduce stress, if nothing else. The objectives of hydrotherapy are to increase range of motion; relieve painful muscle spasms; relax muscles, tendons, and ligaments; and improve overall wellbeing. However, in an analysis published online April 11, 2015, in the *Cochrane Database of Systematic Reviews*, researchers concluded, "Overall evidence is insufficient to show that balneotherapy is more effective than no treatment, that one type of bath is more effective than another, or that one type of bath is more effective than mudpacks, exercise, or relaxation therapy."

Mind/body techniques

Naturally, chronic pain from arthritis can cause distress and depression, and affect your mental state, but evidence also shows that your mental outlook can influence your perception of pain and your ability to cope with arthritis and other pain conditions. One study found that people with depression and mild-to-moderate knee OA reported an increase in pain even when X-rays did not indicate significant joint damage.

Mind/body techniques include biofeedback, meditation, and other relaxation therapies, such as massage. Specialists who treat pain from arthritis and other diseases often use these techniques either alone or in combination with medication.

Massage therapy

Therapeutic massage can loosen tight tissues around an arthritic joint, prompt the body to release natural painkilling endorphins, and increase blood flow to aid in healing. The therapy tends to work best when done regularly—you may need weekly sessions for several weeks before you scale back to monthly treatments. A 2014 study found that hour-long massage sessions given two or three times a week significantly improved chronic neck pain over four weeks, compared to shorter sessions.

Massage cannot correct structural problems caused by arthritis, and results vary from person to person. Still, when combined with medical and physical therapy, massage therapy may ease pain and improve function in arthritis patients.

Massage therapy encompasses an assortment of styles, some better for arthritis than others. Deep-tissue massage may create inflammation and leave you too sore to move freely, so gentler massage and touch therapies may be more appropriate, especially for older adults with osteoporosis.

Biofeedback

During a biofeedback session, devices monitor several of your body functions and use gauges to show you what success you're having at learning to control and lower these functions. The treatment may not provide much help for knee arthritis, but it can be effective where muscle tightness plays a role, especially in the neck or back.

Meditation and mindfulness

Because stress is believed to be associated with flare-ups in several forms of arthritis, including RA, meditation is often used to help reduce anxiety and chronic pain. It helps you beat stress by relaxing your breathing, lowering your heart rate, and reducing any muscle tension.

Some pain experts also recommend mindfulness training, in which patients become aware of thoughts and sensations that may be correlated with anxiety, without stressing about ways to fix them. The treatment is designed to help patients manage anxiety, which can exacerbate pain conditions such as arthritis.

Diet and arthritis

The link between diet and arthritis is tenuous at best. A review of the scientific literature found that no conclusive evidence exists to show that particular foods make RA symptoms flare up or subside. In the review, only a Mediterranean diet (emphasizing fruits, vegetables, nuts, and olive oil) and a fasting/lacto-vegetarian eating plan (fasting for seven to 10 days, followed by a lacto-vegetarian diet that included some milk products) seemed to reduce RA-related pain, but they did not improve stiffness or physical function. Results from other diets were "unclear." The reviewers also noted that the safety of any diet requiring the elimination of whole food groups is questionable.

Scientists have reported that one dietary habit—eating high amounts of salt—may contribute to autoimmune diseases, such as RA, by sparking production of a type of cell linked with autoimmune diseases and inflammation. For instance, a 2014 study found a link between high sodium consumption and increased risk of RA in smokers, but not non-smokers. Although it's too early to tell if a low-salt diet may reduce the risk of RA, eating a low-sodium diet is generally good for your overall health and has been shown to have beneficial effects on blood pressure and cardiovascular disease prevention. Experts recommend limiting sodium consumption to no more than 2,300 mg a day—1,500 mg a day for people over age 51 and others at higher risk of cardiovascular disease is recommended by the American Heart Association.

The nightshade diet

Potatoes, eggplant, tomatoes, and green peppers all belong to a family of plants known as nightshades. Some people find that eating members of this plant group leads to a buildup of toxins that can make their arthritis worse by interfering with an enzyme in their muscles and causing pain. However, there is no scientific evidence to support this belief, and by cutting out these vegetables you miss out on good sources of vitamin C.

Gout and diet

Gout is one of the few forms of arthritis in which diet seems to play a genuine role. Some studies have found that drinking water

Wine may help your knees, but beer may be harmful

Drinking wine may lower your risk of developing knee osteoarthritis (OA), while drinking beer may increase it, recent research suggests. The study included 1,001 people with knee OA, 993 with hip OA, and 933 arthritis-free controls, all of whom answered questionnaires about their alcohol consumption. Compared with abstainers, people who drank four to six glasses of wine per week were 45 percent less likely to develop knee OA, while those who drank seven or more glasses of wine reduced their risk by 52 percent. (The researchers identified no association between wine consumption and hip OA.) The news wasn't so good for heavy beer drinkers: Compared to non-drinkers, those who consumed 20 or more half-pints of beer per week were about twice as likely to develop knee or hip OA.

Arthritis Research & Therapy, February 2015

or skim milk may help prevent gout attacks, while consuming meat, seafood, and sugary drinks and fruits may increase gout risk.

Gout occurs when uric acid crystals are deposited in the joints. Uric acid forms when the body metabolizes substances called purines, which are found in a variety of foods, so if you have gout, your doctor will recommend a diet that limits purine-rich foods and beverages. If you are at increased risk of gout or already have it:

▶ Avoid high-purine foods and beverages: Organ meats (liver, kidneys, hearts, sweetbreads, brains); game meats (squirrel, venison); anchovies, fish eggs, sardines, herring, mackerel, trout, cod, haddock, scallops and mussels; veal, turkey, gravy, broth, bouillon, and consommé; and beer and distilled spirits.

▶ Limit moderate-purine foods to occasional consumption: Asparagus, cauliflower, green peas, kidney beans, lima beans, spinach, and mushrooms; beef, ham, chicken, duck, and pork; crab, oysters, and shrimp; oats and oatmeal, wheat germ and bran, and whole-grain breads and cereals.

Here's to your joint health

Although consumption of alcoholic beverages can increase uric acid levels and precipitate gout attacks, and alcohol misuse may increase the risk of complications after joint-replacement surgery, moderate imbibing may have some beneficial effects against RA. In a 2014 study, researchers reported that women who consumed about one alcoholic drink per day were 22 percent less likely to develop RA compared to teetotalers, while women who drank beer two to four times a week were 31 percent less likely than non-beer drinkers to develop RA. However, too much beer may have a negative effect on knee OA, a recent study suggests (see Box 5-8, "Wine may help your knees, but beer may be harmful"). Experts do not recommend that teetotalers start drinking alcohol to gain health benefits, but if you already drink moderately, you might be helping your joints, studies suggest.

Another beverage, milk, also may do your body—specifically your joints—good. A 2014 study found that women who regularly drank fat-free or low-fat milk experienced slower progression of knee OA; however, eating high amounts of cheese hastened the disease's advance.

Green tea to the rescue

Tea—whether green or black—contains an abundance of antioxidants, and a few preliminary studies have suggested that drinking tea may reduce inflammation or slow cartilage breakdown.

For instance, one study found that epigallocatechin-3-gallate, a powerful anti-inflammatory compound in green tea, may suppress a number of cytokines that have been implicated in causing damage to cartilage and subchondral bone in OA. In an earlier study, epigallocatechin-3-gallate inhibited the production of several molecules in the immune system that contribute to inflammation and joint damage in people with RA. However, these findings need validation from further studies.

Gluten-free vegan diet

Health fanatics aren't the only people who can benefit from this eating plan, which is free of gluten, a protein found in animal products such as meat, cheese and eggs, as well as in wheat, oats, rye, barley, and other grains. One study found that the diet may help protect RA patients against heart attacks and stroke.

Earlier research found that people who consumed a gluten-free vegan diet for a minimum of nine months were more likely than those who ate a non-vegan diet to experience at least a 20 percent improvement in RA symptoms.

Diet's true impact still questionable

Research has yet to prove conclusively that one type of food increases or reduces the risk of OA or RA, or improves or worsens symptoms. Regardless, it certainly doesn't hurt to eat a balanced diet rich in fruits, vegetables, legumes, nuts, and fish— all of which have anti-inflammatory properties. Following this eating plan may benefit your heart and overall health, as well as your joints.

On the flip side, minimize or avoid consumption of processed foods, added sugars and saturated/trans fats. These foods may promote inflammation and also contribute to obesity, a well-known risk factor for arthritis.

Overall, if you notice that a particular food seems to worsen your arthritis, you might try eliminating it for a short period of time to see if your symptoms improve. But note that interpreting

BOX 5-9

Possible impact of arthritis medications on dietary needs

An often-overlooked issue is the effect osteo-arthritis medications can have on your nutritional needs. Some medications can throw off your electrolyte balance, and you may need to adjust your diet to restore it. Those who take prednisone (or other corticosteroids) to treat rheumatoid arthritis tend to lose potassium and retain excess sodium. To offset this, you should eat more fruits (bananas or raisins) to add potassium, and cut back on salt to lower your sodium levels. Prednisone can also lead to thinning of the bones (osteopenia and osteoporosis), so you may need to start taking a calcium and vitamin D supplement. Methotrexate, another drug taken to manage rheumatoid arthritis, can lower your folic acid levels. To compensate, take either a multivitamin (minimum of 0.4 mg of folic acid) or eat foods rich in this B vitamin, such as liver, fresh green vegetables, fruit, and/or fortified breakfast cereals.

the impact of a diet or use of a supplement on your arthritis can be tricky because arthritis—especially RA—goes through periods of spontaneous remission and flare-up, independent of anything you might do. These remissions can last for a few days, weeks, or months, so if you begin your dietary experiment at the same time your arthritis goes into remission, it's easy to mistakenly attribute any improvement to the dietary change instead of to chance (see Box 5-9, "Possible impact of arthritis medications on dietary needs").

Transcutaneous electrical nerve stimulation (TENS)

Transcutaneous electrical nerve stimulation (TENS) uses low-level electrical pulses that travel quickly along the nerves to your brain, blocking slower-moving pain messages. In the process, they also trigger the release of your body's natural pain-controlling endorphins. TENS does not provide immediate pain relief, but requires a week or more of daily sessions before you will experience significant benefits.

Once reserved primarily for use by physical therapists, TENS units have been simplified—some have even been incorporated into knee braces—and are now widely available to the public. Some patients use TENS regularly, others only as needed, for about 10 to 15 minutes per treatment session.

Overall, studies of the use of TENS to treat arthritis and back pain have produced conflicting results. American Academy of Neurology guidelines do not recommend TENS for chronic lower back pain, although the American College of Rheumatology conditionally recommends that patients with knee OA be instructed in the use of TENS.

Magnet therapy

Electromagnets have been used in conventional medicine for several years to speed the healing of fractured bones and to map areas of the brain. Experimentally, they have been used to treat fibromyalgia, chronic pain, and headaches. However, most of the magnets found in shoe inserts, belts, mattress pads, and cushions as "health aids" are static magnets, and there is no credible scientific evidence to back their use.

Magnets are generally safe, but manufacturers don't recommend them for pregnant women, those with pacemakers, defibrillators, or insulin pumps, individuals who use a patch that delivers medication through the skin, or anyone who has had an aneurysm clipped. The National Institutes of Health reports that people who benefit from magnets usually see results quickly. If you buy one, make sure it has a 30-day return policy in case it doesn't work.

Dimethyl sulfoxide (DMSO)

Dimethyl sulfoxide (DMSO) is believed to have anti-inflammatory properties and can be used as a topical treatment that proponents say may relieve swelling and pain from arthritis when rubbed into the skin near a sore joint. Some studies have suggested a benefit from both DMSO and a related oral supplement, methylsulfonylmethane (MSM) when it comes to easing pain associated with knee OA—however, a review of the medical literature concluded that the available evidence prevents any definitive conclusions from being drawn about the effectiveness of either supplement for this purpose. Still, DMSO, an organic byproduct of wood pulp processing, is a component of a topical diclofenac prescription product (Pennsaid) approved for treating knee OA, and it is found in some non-prescription products. DMSO is also used as an industrial solvent available in hardware stores—use of this industrial-strength form as a topical treatment may pose health risks, and should be avoided.

WHAT YOU CAN DO

About half of knee OA cases in the U.S. could be avoided, and more than 111,000 knee replacements could be averted each year if obesity were removed as a risk factor.

Medications, injections, supplements, surgery. They're helpful treatments that have provided pain relief and improved function for millions of arthritis patients. But perhaps nothing can do as much for your joints as the things you can do yourself—namely, exercise and weight management.

The hard truth is that by remaining sedentary and packing on pounds, you're putting your joints at risk of arthritis damage. And if you already have arthritis, inactivity and obesity can add to your pain, weaken your joints, and further erode your quality of life. Fortunately, by augmenting medical and surgical treatments with lifestyle changes, support devices, and simple coping strategies, you can function better with arthritis and keep it from seriously disrupting your life.

Exercise

Exercise is an important part of any comprehensive arthritis treatment plan because it improves joint mobility, muscle strength, and overall conditioning, and helps you maintain a healthy weight (see Box 6-1, "Types of exercise"). It also releases endorphins: the body's natural painkillers, which can help you feel good in general.

Additionally, staying active may improve your level of pain and functioning and boost your overall health, research suggests (see Box 6-2, "Exercise, manual therapy help with OA"). One study found that knee osteoarthritis (OA) patients who were physically active—even if they didn't meet guidelines calling for 150 minutes of physical activity a week—showed improvements that translated into about 10 to 20 more days of good health in a year, compared to their sedentary counterparts. In another study, researchers found that among 1,788 obese people (average age 67) with or at high risk of knee OA, few of the participants who walked more than 3,000 steps a day developed functional limitations two years later, and that walking 6,000 steps a day appeared to be the threshold that separated people

BOX 6-1

Types of exercise

Arthritis exercises come in three types:

- **Stretching or range-of-motion exercise:** Exercises that help you regain more normal joint movement and relieve stiffness. In these, you move a joint as far as it will comfortably go, and then slowly learn to stretch it a bit farther to increase mobility and range of motion.

- **Strength or resistance exercise:** Exercises that help build muscle strength and sometimes size. In these, you use either the weight of your own body or other weights to tone and strengthen your muscles and stabilize weak joints.

- **Aerobic or endurance exercise:** Exercises that improve cardiovascular fitness, build stamina, and help with weight control. These typically last 15 minutes or more and involve major muscle groups.

who developed functional limitations from those who did not. The researchers suggested an initial minimum goal of 3,000 steps (about 1½ miles) per day, gradually increasing to 6,000 steps (about three miles) per day, for people with knee OA.

Other evidence suggests that taking part in exercises that improve hip strength and mobility may help patients with hip OA delay, or even avoid, the need for total hip replacement. In a study of 108 people with symptomatic hip OA, researchers concluded that, compared with education about hip OA alone, exercise therapy reduced the need for hip replacement by 44 percent, and delayed the need for surgery by nearly two years.

Exercise and strength training are of particular importance to rheumatoid arthritis (RA) patients, because a large number of them have only the minimum strength needed to handle a variety of daily activities, such as walking, rising from a seated position, and climbing stairs. Any further decline in strength, even if small, could put them below the threshold needed to carry out these activities and threaten their ability to maintain an independent lifestyle.

For those with OA, exercise combined with weight loss can lead to dramatic improvement. One study found that losing just five percent of total body weight within a 20-week period should be enough for overweight or obese people with knee OA to feel and function better. Exercise also can help strengthen your hips and shoulders. (See pages 104-108 for easy exercises to relieve pain and keep shoulders, hands, hips, and ankles strong and flexible.)

Exercise guidelines

Exercise guidelines from the American College of Sports Medicine include recommendations tailored for adults over age 65. Among the recommendations:

▶ Do moderately intense aerobic exercise 30 to 60 minutes a day for five days a week, or vigorously intense exercise 20 to 30 minutes a day for three days a week. With moderate-intensity exercise, you should still be able to talk to the person next to you while exercising, but not so with vigorous exercise.

▶ Do eight to 10 strength-training exercises (eight to 12 repetitions of each), at fairly light to mildly strenuous exertion, on two

NEW FINDING   BOX 6-2

Exercise, manual therapy help with OA

In a study involving 206 people (average age 66) with hip or knee osteoarthritis, those who added sustained exercise physical therapy or manual therapy (joint mobilization) to standard medical care gained more benefits than those given medical care alone. The participants were assigned to receive physical therapy, manual therapy, a combination of both, or standard medical care alone. Those in the therapy groups received seven sessions scheduled over nine weeks, another two at four months, and a final session at 13 months. At the end of a two-year follow-up period, all the participants in the therapy groups showed greater improvements in pain, stiffness, and physical function compared to those who received only standard medical care.

American College of Rheumatology Annual Meeting, November 2014

or more nonconsecutive days of the week. Rest one or two seconds between each repetition.

» **Do balance exercises if you're at risk of falling.** Try standing on one foot while holding onto a chair. Or, try a tai chi class taught by a certified instructor. Don't attempt balance exercises for the first time when you're alone.

» **Do 10 minutes of flexibility exercises (stretching) at least two days a week.** Do your stretches after your other exercises, or independent of them.

If you have arthritis, your physician and/or an exercise professional can help customize an exercise regimen tailored to your individual capabilities. Develop a physical activity plan that addresses each type of exercise, how to monitor your activity, and how to re-evaluate your exercise regimen as your health status changes.

Stretching, or range-of-motion, exercises

In range-of-motion exercises, or stretches, you condition your joints to become more flexible by slowly and gently bending and straightening them as far as they will go, but not to the point of discomfort. Over time, and with repetition, a joint's comfort range can gradually be broadened and, in some cases, approach normal.

Strength or resistance exercises

Whether done on a mat, in a pool, with free weights or weight machines, resistance or strength exercises challenge your body to build stronger, larger muscles that give you better posture and help you move your joints more easily. For example, research suggests that strength-training exercises that target the large quadriceps muscles on the front of your thigh may help combat knee OA. Resistance exercises also may help people with hip OA reduce pain, improve mobility, and, possibly, slow the course of their disease, according to one study. And because muscle tissue burns more calories than fat tissue, having larger muscles is a way to turn your overall metabolism up a notch and more easily keep your weight in check.

Using water for resistance

Water can provide a gentle form of resistance known as water therapy, hydrotherapy, or aqua therapy. For those with moderate-to-severe arthritis, exercising in a pool at the local YMCA or health club helps because the water not only warms your joints but helps support your body, reducing the weight on your spine, legs and feet as you move. Swimming isn't required, as these exercises may be done while sitting in a shallow pool.

You also might try spinning classes in which you ride a partially submerged stationary bike. Instructors claim the water workouts burn up to 600 calories an hour, and because the bike is underwater, the impact on your bones and joints is lessened. While your legs are pumping through the water, you work your upper body with the help of small hand weights or by moving your arms in a swimming motion.

Aerobic or endurance exercise

If your overall health and fitness level are good enough, aerobic or endurance exercises should be added to stretching and resistance exercises.

In endurance exercise, you work the large muscles of your body for an extended period of time, with the goal of gradually increasing the stamina of your heart, lungs, and overall cardiovascular system. This exercise trains your body to use oxygen better, improves overall circulation, and helps you develop stronger muscles. It also is a proven method for weight control, especially when combined with a healthy diet.

Talk to your doctor or therapist to determine what starting level of endurance exercise is right for you. Even if you start out with just five minutes of sustained exercise, you should be able to gradually build up to 30 minutes a day. Your pace should be comfortable, yet challenging, allowing you enough breath to have a normal conversation. Ideally, you want to do 30 minutes of endurance exercises daily—all at once or in three 10-minute sessions—at least five days a week. Warm up with a low-intensity form of your exercise for at least five to 10 minutes before each workout, and then cool down with another five minutes of range-of-motion movements afterward.

Although exercise, in general, is an effective tool for managing your arthritis, in some instances, it can do more harm than good (see Box 6-3, "Danger signs during or after exercise"). Be wary of exercises that require bending forward (sit-ups, toe touches), that

BOX 6-3

Danger signs during or after exercise

If you notice any of the following during or after your workout, give your doctor a call.

- Unusual or persistent fatigue
- Sharp or increased pain
- Increased weakness
- Decreased range of motion
- Increased joint swelling
- Continuing pain (lasting at least two hours)

BOX 6-4

Running may protect against knee OA

Running or jogging not only doesn't increase your risk of developing knee osteoarthritis (OA), but it also may protect you from developing it in the first place, a recent study suggests. Researchers examined data on 2,683 people, average age about 64, nearly one-third of whom reported that they'd been runners at some point in their lives. The participants were surveyed about their exercise habits at different time periods, underwent knee X-rays, and completed assessments of their knee pain. Those who were runners, regardless of the age when they ran, had a lower prevalence of knee pain, signs of OA on X-ray, and symptomatic OA than non-runners. Non-elite running at any time in life does not appear detrimental, and may be protective against symptomatic knee OA, the researchers concluded.

American College of Rheumatology Annual Meeting, November 2014

BOX 6-5

Use caution when jogging

Some doctors recommend that those who have had a severe joint injury or are genetically predisposed to arthritis avoid jogging altogether, while others suggest you just need to be more cautious before you lace up your running shoes. Here's how to be more cautious:

- Run on more joint-forgiving surfaces, such as dirt or a padded track, rather than on asphalt or concrete.
- Replace your shoes every 400 miles, before the built-in shock absorption begins to degrade.
- Run no more often than every other day, to give joints time to rest, repair and recover.

increase the likelihood of falls (step aerobics, anything done on a slippery floor), or that jar the spine (running on a hard surface, jumping, or high-impact aerobics).

It's a common belief that the impact of running or jogging can contribute to knee or hip OA or exacerbate its symptoms. Running places excessive stress on the leg joints, resulting in forces of more than seven times your body weight on the knees and five times your body weight on the hips. Yet, a 2014 study suggests that running may, in fact, reduce the risk of knee OA (see Box 6-4, "Running may protect against knee OA"). Nevertheless, if you run or jog, it's important to take precautions to minimize the effects on your knees or hips (see Box 6-5, "Use caution when jogging").

Sports smarts

Just because we age, it doesn't mean we have to stop taking part in the sports we love. But it does mean we need to be a bit smarter about the activities we choose and, in some cases, adjust our technique or equipment in order to reduce the stress on aging joints. Here are some sport-specific tips that should help you compete, despite having arthritis.

Golf

According to the Arthritis Foundation, swinging a golf club can enhance the range of motion in your shoulders, as well as improve balance and overall coordination. However, be careful on the links if you've recently had a knee replacement. Although golf typically is considered a low-impact activity, one study found that a full golf swing can take its toll on new artificial knees, generating high forces in the forward knee and less on the opposite knee.

To make things a bit easier on your hands, wrists, and other joints:

- Use clubs with lightweight graphite shafts.
- Switch to a lower-compression ball.
- Use perimeter-weighted clubs.
- Wear wrist braces or gloves on both hands to better stabilize your joints.
- Build up the thickness of your grips with tape to ease stress on hands and fingers.

- Wear spikeless or other comfortable shoes.
- Afterward, take a warm bath or shower to relax.

Swimming

Water exercise is often a part of arthritis therapy, since it helps take the load off joints even while you put them through a workout. Modify your technique to fit your needs:

- Cut back on total distance, but swim the shorter distance at a faster rate.
- Pick a stroke and intensity level that are comfortable. The breaststroke, rather than freestyle, might be better if you have arthritis in your upper body.
- Include some resistance exercises that help strengthen your rotator cuffs and the muscles that stabilize the shoulder blades.

Tennis

Play doubles instead of singles to cut back on the need for the frequent starting, stopping, and changes of direction that makes tennis so taxing on the knees.

Skiing

Switch to somewhat less challenging slopes to cut back on the range of motion required. Mix in some cross-country skiing, which is easier on the joints and probably closer to home.

Weight control

Being overweight is one of the most important factors in the development of osteoarthritis (OA), and the added wear and tear placed on your joints may be only one factor in a complex inter-action between obesity and OA. Researchers are learning that increased weight not only places added stress on your knees and hips, but also harms your joints on a metabolic level. Fat (or adipose) cells and tissue aren't just inactive energy storage centers, as once believed—rather, they act like an endocrine organ, producing inflammatory substances that damage artic-ular cartilage. Studies have found that obese patients have an increased risk of OA even in non-weight-bearing joints, such as the hand.

Sustained weight loss relieves knee OA pain

A recent study suggests that obese patients with knee osteoarthritis (OA) who lose weight and maintain that weight loss may reduce their OA symptoms. The study included 192 obese patients age 50 and older with knee OA, who underwent a 16-week intensive dietary weight-loss program. Then, to maintain their weight loss, the participants were randomized to a dietary intervention, knee-exercise program, or no formal intervention for another 52 weeks. All of the participants who sustained their weight loss, regardless of how they did it, experienced improvements in pain and other knee OA symptoms after one year, the researchers reported.

Arthritis Care & Research, November 2014

Increased weight also can make your arthritis symptoms worse. Therefore, you can help relieve arthritis symptoms by reducing your weight (see Box 6-6, "Sustained weight loss relieves knee OA pain").

Evidence suggests that weight loss actually may prevent knee OA. In a 2013 report, experts noted that about half of knee OA cases in the U.S. could be avoided and more than 111,000 knee replacements could be averted each year if obesity were removed as a risk factor.

Though losing weight takes a great deal of willpower, it's one of the best ways to ease the strain on an arthritic spine, hip, knee, or foot. For those with knee arthritis, each pound of weight loss reduces the stress on the knee by four to eight pounds. Lose 10 pounds and you could reduce the stress on your knees by as much as 80 pounds.

So, you don't have to lose lots of weight to have a big effect on your arthritis risk. One study suggests that losing enough weight to move from the obese category to the overweight category, or from overweight to normal (a loss of perhaps 10 to 20 pounds) could reduce a man's risk of knee OA by 21 percent, and a woman's by 33 percent. Those facing possible knee-replacement surgery sometimes find that losing weight allows them to delay the need for the procedure, while research suggests that being obese may increase the risk of complications and poor outcomes after hip replacement and other orthopaedic surgery.

Calculate your body mass index (BMI)

Doctors rely on a measure called the body mass index (BMI) to figure out if you are obese and need to lose weight. To calculate your own BMI, start with your body weight, multiply it by 703, and then divide that by your height in inches squared. A BMI between 18.5 and 24.9 is considered normal, 25 to 29.9 is overweight, and 30 or higher is obese.

Drink plenty of water

For people with arthritis, especially those who may be overweight, drinking lots of water has special importance. Your cartilage, which is largely liquid, softens the impact of walking by squeezing out some of its water into the synovial space. So drinking plenty of water is key to keeping your spongy cartilage hydrated and soft, step after step, even if you are carrying a few extra pounds. Most experts agree that you should drink at least five 8-ounce glasses of water a day.

Know your resting metabolic rate

In order to effectively manage your weight, you first need to know how many calories you normally burn at rest. However, this rate, known as the resting metabolic rate, or RMR, can vary widely from person to person and play a big part in how you customize a dietary plan to suit your needs. Fortunately, a widely available handheld breath test (the BodyGem) can give you the answer in 10 minutes. Once you know your RMR, then you know not to restrict your daily calories any lower than this number, or your body will go into starvation mode and lower its metabolism to protect itself. Generally, you want to aim for a daily calorie limit that is 1.2 to 1.7 times your RMR, depending upon your normal activity level.

Improve your coping skills

The pain of arthritis can get in the way of many day-to-day activities. For each of these activities and more, you can take steps to get the job done easier, and therapists are ready to show you how.

Occupational therapists

Occupational therapists can show you how to modify your office and home, as well as your own movements, in order to reduce the motions that aggravate your joints. Their guidance includes providing splints for your hands or wrists and recommending assistive devices to aid in tasks such as driving, bathing, dressing, housekeeping, and certain work activities.

Knowing when to rest

One way to reduce both pain and inflammation from arthritis is rest. If multiple joints are involved and fatigue is a problem, as is common with rheumatoid arthritis, then bed rest can be helpful. People with RA may find they need more sleep than usual, particularly during a flare-up. For those with discomfort in just a few joints (as is typical of osteoarthritis), splints and other supports can bring relief.

BOX 6-7

Splints, braces, and other mechanical aids

Braces, splints, shoe inserts and other assistive devices may help ease some symptoms of arthritis, and help you function better with it. They are used to temporarily support or stabilize a joint, but should not be seen as a long-term solution (see Box 6-7, "Bracing guidelines"). They are usually made from light-weight metal, leather, elastic, foam, and/or moldable plastic with Velcro straps.

Knees

If you have knee arthritis, your doctor may prescribe braces until you have sufficiently strengthened the muscles around the knee through exercise. Braces can support your knee and reduce excessive loading on an arthritic joint, but how effective they are remains unclear (see Box 6-8, "Knee brace may ease OA pain"). The most basic type is a one-piece sleeve made out of elastic rubber (neoprene) that fits snugly around the knee. These braces, available over the counter, warm and compress the knee, providing moderate support for people with mild knee arthritis.

For more severe arthritis affecting one part of the joint, consider a custom-fit unloader brace, a semi-rigid device made of plastic, foam, and hinged steel struts on each side to limit lateral movement.

Talk to your doctor or an orthopaedic specialist about knee braces and which type is right for you. You may need to see an orthotist, who specializes in fitting custom braces. The specialist also may provide you with shoe inserts, or foot orthotics, which may help with knee arthritis pain.

Feet and ankles

Devices ranging from an ankle brace or semi-rigid foot orthotic to wedge inserts, rocker soles, and customized plastic orthotics, may help improve balance and normalize walking patterns affected by ankle OA. Similarly, a podiatrist may provide orthotics or recommend special shoes to help with foot arthritis.

Wrists and hands

If you have an arthritic wrist, your doctor or therapist may recommend occasional use of a wrist splint to immobilize the joint and prevent the bones from rubbing together. Simple neoprene splints may help patients with milder pain and functional limitations, but custom-molded splints may be better for people with more severe arthritis. Some splints immobilize the hand, while others allow movement. Splinting also may be helpful if you have arthritis at the base of the thumb.

Elbows

Braces can maintain range of motion in the elbow and ease pain. Braces that support the back of the elbow are recommended for people who plan to use them during activity, while a brace that supports the front of the elbow may be more comfortable at night.

Other mechanical aids

A wide variety of devices is available to help support and protect joints:

- **Shock-absorbing soles** in sneakers or orthopedic shoes can help in daily activities and during gentle exercise.
- **Heel wedges** in the shoes can sometimes even help patients avoid knee replacement surgery.
- A **neck brace** or **corset** may relieve back pain.
- A **firm mattress** also often proves beneficial.
- In extreme cases of back pain, lying in **traction** might rarely be used.
- **Canes, crutches or walkers** offer benefits to patients with advanced arthritis. In fact, one study found that using a cane reduced knee adduction (the collapsing of the knee toward the midline of the body), and actually may slow the progression of knee OA.

Coping in the kitchen

A variety of tools has evolved to help those with arthritis cope in the kitchen. Though these tools may be more expensive than the standard tools found in most kitchens, the investment might be worthwhile if it helps those with arthritis enjoy a nutritious diet. Here are some tips for choosing new kitchen equipment or replacing utensils and small appliances:

Knee brace may ease OA pain

Use of a valgus knee brace can help improve pain and function in patients with osteoarthritis on the inside (medial compartment) of the knee joint, according to a recent study. After reviewing data from six randomized studies that included 445 patients (ages 34 to 73), researchers found that compared to no brace, use of a valgus brace resulted in moderate improvements in pain and function. When compared to use of another orthotic device, use of the brace provided small, but statistically significant, benefits in terms of pain, but not function, the study found.

Arthritis Care & Research, April 2015

- **Easy-to-grip handles:** Look for utensils that have larger, easy-to-grip, non-slip handles.
- **Higher openers:** Have your jar or can opener mounted on the underside of an upper cabinet to make reaching and using it easier.
- **Rolling cutter:** Consider a rolling, pizza-style cutter or rocker-cutter to relieve stress on your hand and wrist. Look for other tools that have handles set at 90 degrees from the working surface.
- **Use both hands:** When working with larger pans or skillets, use a pair of mitt-like potholders so you can use both hands.
- **Make cleanup easier:** Use foil, disposable baking pans, and nonstick sprays to make cleaning up easier.

Choose simpler recipes

If your hand or wrist movement is impaired by arthritis, ease the load by rethinking your meal-preparation strategy and choosing recipes that are easier to make. Try picking recipes with no more than five ingredients, as well as those that include ingredients that are easier to prepare.

Coping with housework

To divide and conquer is the best way to approach the various chores that can otherwise seem daunting when thought of, or attempted, all at once.

- **Break projects into reasonable pieces:** If you have lots of chores on your to-do list, sort them by highest to lowest priority, and try just to get those at the top done first.
- **Group together:** Since using the stairs takes lots of energy, conserve yours by grouping your chores by floor or area of the house.
- **Alternate by type:** Try to alternate chores that require standing and sitting, to give your joints a break. Follow a round of dish washing by sitting down and folding laundry, for example.
- **Lighten your load:** If you find yourself dragging cleaning tools and supplies all over the house, put duplicate sets of cleaning tools on every floor.

Coping in the garden

An array of methods and tools can help you take care of your yard and garden, while easing the strain on your hands, back, knees, and other joints.

- Sit, don't bend: Ease the stress on your back by sitting on a garden bench or overturned bucket when working. A long pole or broom handle can help you make holes for planting.
- Keep plants within reach: Reduce the need to bend by using raised flowerbeds and containers. Use more window boxes and trellises to keep things within easier reach.
- Modified tools: Most garden stores carry ergonomic tools with smart designs that are easier on your hands and wrists.
- Easy access to tools: Keep commonly used tools nearby on hooks or shelves to reduce the need to bend and sort through crowded cupboards.
- Lighten the load: Use more mulch and other cover around your plants to keep the weeds and the workload down.
- Timing is everything: Weed your garden after it's been watered or after a rain, to reduce the energy needed to pull out weeds.

Shoe logic

Bony osteoarthritic spurs at the base of the big toe may widen the foot and make wearing wider shoes necessary. Any attempt at wearing pointed or high-heeled shoes will be particularly uncomfortable.

Also, the types of shoes you wear may affect your risk of knee OA, according to one study. Researchers found that clogs and stability shoes caused significantly higher loading of the knees, while walking shoes and flip-flops resulted in lower loading (similar to that when walking barefoot), thereby allowing a more natural foot motion and flexibility that was helpful in slowing the progression of knee OA.

Those with rheumatoid arthritis may develop tender calluses and ulcerations at the ball of the foot. Though these sometimes require surgery, you can take some of the pressure off by having your shoes modified, with a leather strap or wedge added to the sole of your shoe, just behind the arch of the foot. And to reduce the need for bending when putting on your shoes, try a long-handled shoehorn.

Tips on finding comfortable shoes

When shopping for shoes:

▶ Buy shoes late in the day. Feet swell as the day progresses.

▶ Don't select shoes just by the size marked inside the shoe. Sizes vary among brands and styles.

▶ Your feet expand while bearing weight, so stand while your feet are being measured.

▶ There should be at least a half-inch space between your longest toe and the tip of the shoe.

▶ Make sure the shoes fit in the store. If they don't feel good in the store, they probably won't feel good at home.

Get into a good position

Using good posture and getting your body into the right position at home, work, and play keeps your bones and joints in proper alignment, allowing muscles to work more efficiently. As a result, you'll help reduce the stress and wear on joints that may already be a bit sore from arthritis.

At the office

Sit down to do a job instead of standing. Change position often, since staying in one position for a long time tends to increase stiffness and pain. If you carry a briefcase or purse, use a shoulder strap instead of your hand.

At home

Use proper body mechanics to get in and out of a car, chair, or tub, as well as for lifting objects (see Box 6-9, "Lift smart"). When lifting, use your strongest joints and muscles to reduce the stress on smaller joints. In the kitchen, lift dishes with both palms rather than with your fingers, and carry heavy loads in your arms instead of with your hands.

Choosing the right chair

The right chair can making living with arthritis a lot easier (see Box 6-10, "Sit smart"). To find one that won't put undue stress on already sore hips, knees, or wrists, here are a few guidelines:

▶ Firmer is better: You want a seat cushion firm enough so you

BOX 6-9

LIFT SMART

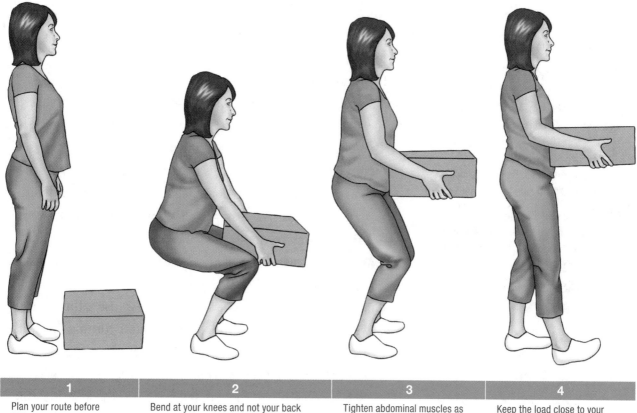

1	2	3	4
Plan your route before lifting.	Bend at your knees and not your back when you begin, keeping shoulders upright.	Tighten abdominal muscles as you lift.	Keep the load close to your body.

can push off and stable enough to put your back in a position of consistent lumbar support.

▶ **Feet on the floor:** Your feet should be able to rest flat on the floor when seated in an upright position, all the way back. If not, your lumbar spine will lack support.

▶ **Armrests matter:** To gain leverage when getting up, look for armrests that extend slightly forward from the front of the chair and offer a good, secure grip for arthritic hands.

▶ **Test drive it:** Spend at least 20 minutes in a new easy chair before buying it, and make sure to get a money-back guarantee in case you need to return it after a few days or weeks.

Sleep smart

For arthritis patients, the most important features of a mattress are surface firmness and how that surface accommodates gentle changes in sleeping position during the night.

BOX 6-10

Sit smart

- Get an adjustable chair with lumbar support, and sit all the way back.

- Sit with legs at a 90-degree angle and feet flat on the floor.

- Sit close enough to your desk to use the keyboard or mouse without leaning forward.

BOX 6-11

Traveling with arthritis

WHEN FLYING:

- Allow extra time to get to your gate.

- Use curbside check-in. Check your bag if it weighs more than 15 pounds.

- Book an aisle seat so you can stretch your legs and walk around.

WHEN DRIVING:

- Exercise at stoplights. Roll your shoulders, tilt your head from side to side, and stretch your neck.

- If your car has lumbar support, use it; keep the seat far enough back so you can almost fully extend your legs.

- Schedule stops every hour to stretch and avoid stiffness.

The use of a proper mattress is most important for people with arthritis in the large, weight-bearing joints. If you've been sleeping on a surface that's too soft and have been sinking into it, your shoulders, hips, and back will be sore from the unequal pressure that's exerted on them.

When shopping for a mattress:

- Start early: Begin your search for a new mattress as soon as you notice that your pain is at least as bad in the morning as it was when you went to bed the night before.

- Test drive it: Never purchase a mattress that you haven't tried.

- Firmer is better: When in doubt, choose a firmer rather than softer mattress. The firmness allows you to turn over more easily during the night.

- Avoid futons and waterbeds: These are too soft, and waterbeds are too difficult to get in and out of.

- Right sheets: If you prefer a softer mattress, use satin sheets or wear silk nightclothes, which will facilitate turning over with ease.

- Consider memory foam: Mattresses with surfaces made of "memory foam" are popular among those with arthritis, since the material self-adjusts to your shape and weight.

Once you've selected a mattress, positioning is as important as firmness. It should be low enough so that you don't have to leap down out of bed but high enough so that you don't have to bend your knees excessively in order to get into and out of bed.

Coping on the road

Americans are traveling more often and taking more medications than ever, potentially creating a recipe for trouble. But you can avoid problems if you plan ahead. Here are a few suggestions to help you better manage your medications and enjoy your trip (also see Box 6-11, "Traveling with arthritis"):

- Put medications in carry-on luggage: Even when traveling by car, it's best to keep climate-sensitive medications close by, and store them as you do at home. Glove compartments and trunks are not temperature-controlled, and drugs can degrade quickly in humid conditions.

- Pack more medicine: Always pack more than you plan on

taking. If your trip is extended, you'll have enough to last until you return home.

‣ **Carry medications in original, labeled containers:** Keep drugs in separate labeled containers. If you combine them into one container you may not be able to identify them, and could end up taking the wrong medication, missing a dose, or taking the wrong dose.

‣ **Bring bottled water to take medications:** Don't take drugs with coffee, tea, or other hot beverages that can reduce their effectiveness.

‣ **Bring a list:** Bring along a complete list of your medications, as well as phone numbers and email addresses of your doctor and pharmacist. Carry this information separately from your medications in case you lose or misplace them.

‣ **Make sure syringes are labeled:** If your medication requires a syringe, the syringe must have the manufacturer's or pharmacist's label attached. Better yet, ask your doctor for a note explaining your condition and the need for a syringe.

‣ **Plan for time zone changes:** To help you take your meds on schedule, despite trips across several time zones, bring along two watches or clocks—one set to local time, the other to the time back home.

‣ **Be aware of medications that make you light sensitive:** Some drugs (taken for depression, cancer, hypertension, inflammation, and other conditions) can make you more sensitive to sunlight. Make sure you know if you need to cover up or put on extra sunscreen before heading to the beach.

‣ **Be aware of local drug regulations:** Some countries have tighter restrictions than the U.S. on drugs you may be taking.

Better hand health

Few parts of our body play such a key role in how we take part in everyday life, yet the free and easy dexterity of our hands is often taken for granted until the cartilage of the palm, wrist, or finger joints begins to erode and the pain begins (see Box 6-12, "Steps to better hand health").

People with hand-intense occupations and hobbies are more likely to develop early wear and tear, especially if they do a lot of

BOX 6-12

Steps to better hand health

- Take regular breaks from hand-intensive activity.
- Avoid repetitive stresses on your hand joints and extreme or awkward hand postures.
- Use ergonomic tools: they are usually larger, fit more of the hand, and reduce stress on any one area.
- Perform daily hand exercises that involve stretching.

pinching, twisting, or squeezing with their hands. Osteoarthritis of the hands is also more likely in those who've suffered a previous injury, such as a fractured wrist or jammed finger.

Reducing stress on hands

The best defense against hand arthritis is to postpone it as long as possible by reducing the amount of stress you put on the joints of your hands.

▶ **Do things less often:** Reduce how often you use your hands to pinch, grip, or twist. Take more frequent breaks when using your hands in such a manner, or simply cut back on how often you engage in such an activity.

▶ **Alter your tools or technique:** Look for a way to modify your technique or tool so that it takes some of the stress off your hands. Many ergonomic tools can help you redistribute a lot of the stress from the small joints in your hands to your larger, more durable elbow and shoulder joints.

Warm them up to reduce pain

Once you develop osteoarthritis of the hands, the focus is then on how best to manage the pain so that you can continue to use your hands to the fullest. If your hands are most stiff and sore first thing in the morning, use a heating pad or paraffin bath to warm them up. Warmed joints help ease the pain, and will allow for easier range of motion. Warming up your hands is also recommended before taking your hands through any type of stretches that help with flexibility and range of motion.

Stretch, don't squeeze

If you suffer from hand arthritis, stretching your fingers will do the most good—and the least harm (see "Appendix I: Exercises" on page 104). Exercises that involve squeezing a ball or a special grip device can put undue stress on already damaged joints, so don't use such devices without the guidance of a therapist or physician.

CONCLUSION

As you've read in this report, you have a wide assortment of treatments at your disposal to help you cope with arthritis and improve your function.

It takes a joint effort on the part of you, your doctor, and the rest of your healthcare team to find the right strategy to manage the pain of osteoarthritis or send rheumatoid arthritis into remission—all the while preserving the health of your joints. Include on your team a physical therapist, who can work with you to develop an exercise regimen tailored to your individual capabilities, to strengthen and improve the motion of your joints. Seek the services of an occupational therapist to guide you on how to function in daily life despite arthritis. And if conservative efforts no longer provide sufficient relief, consult a surgeon and discuss the array of modern surgical options that are providing relief while affording shorter recovery times and lower risks of complications. In general, weigh the pros and cons of all arthritis treatments, and carefully review all of your options with your physician.

In the end, you are the most important factor in managing arthritis and reducing your risk. By optimizing your weight and staying physically active, you might lower your odds of developing arthritis in the first place, or function better if you have the disease. And, by improving your overall health, you might reduce your reliance on medications, and avoid unwanted side effects.

Use this special report to guide discussions with your healthcare team about the best ways to manage your arthritis. And follow the advice on these pages to keep your joints in motion, improve your overall health, and better cope with the unwanted companion known as arthritis.

HIPS
Easy exercises to keep hips strong and flexible

Healthy hip joints are essential for keeping yourself on the go. These ball-and-socket connections between leg and pelvis are at the center of the action each time you sit, stand, take a step, rotate your leg, or bend at the waist. To make sure these activities remain easy to do, it's important that you keep the muscles around your hip joints strong and flexible. These exercises will help you do this; however, some may not be appropriate if you have hip problems. As a general rule, if you feel pain or stiffness when doing any of these exercises, go easy. If the pain gets worse, stop until you have talked to your doctor or physical therapist.

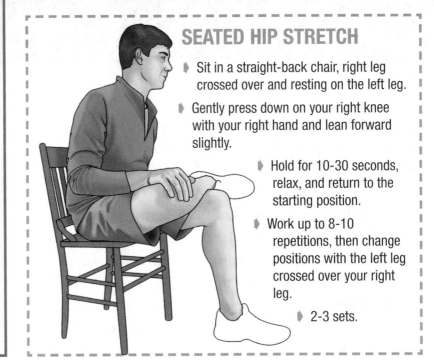

SEATED HIP STRETCH

- Sit in a straight-back chair, right leg crossed over and resting on the left leg.
- Gently press down on your right knee with your right hand and lean forward slightly.
- Hold for 10-30 seconds, relax, and return to the starting position.
- Work up to 8-10 repetitions, then change positions with the left leg crossed over your right leg.
- 2-3 sets.

SIDE LEG LIFTS

- Lie on your left side, right leg resting on your left leg.
- Raise your right leg as high as possible without discomfort, hold for 3-5 seconds, slowly return to the starting position.
- Work up to 8-10 repetitions, 2-3 sets, with each leg.

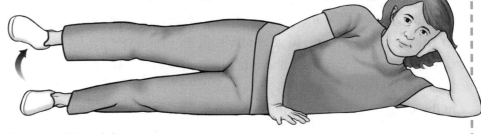

RESISTANCE BAND CLAMSHELLS

- Lie on your left side, right leg on top of the left, knees comfortably bent.
- With a resistance band wrapped around your knees, rotate the right leg up until your leg makes a 90-degree angle to the floor.
- Hold for 1-2 seconds and slowly return to the starting position.
- Change positions and complete the same number of repetitions and sets with the opposite leg, 2-3 sets.

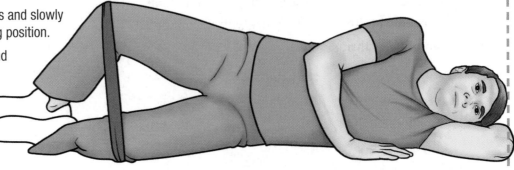

SIDE LEG RAISES

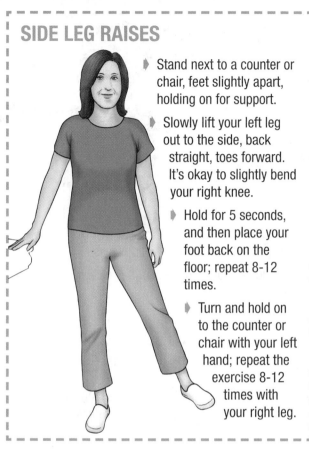

- ▸ Stand next to a counter or chair, feet slightly apart, holding on for support.
- ▸ Slowly lift your left leg out to the side, back straight, toes forward. It's okay to slightly bend your right knee.
  - ▸ Hold for 5 seconds, and then place your foot back on the floor; repeat 8-12 times.
  - ▸ Turn and hold on to the counter or chair with your left hand; repeat the exercise 8-12 times with your right leg.

BACK LEG RAISES

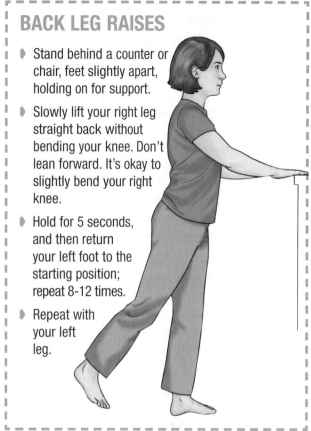

- ▸ Stand behind a counter or chair, feet slightly apart, holding on for support.
- ▸ Slowly lift your right leg straight back without bending your knee. Don't lean forward. It's okay to slightly bend your right knee.
- ▸ Hold for 5 seconds, and then return your left foot to the starting position; repeat 8-12 times.
- ▸ Repeat with your left leg.

HIP FLEXION

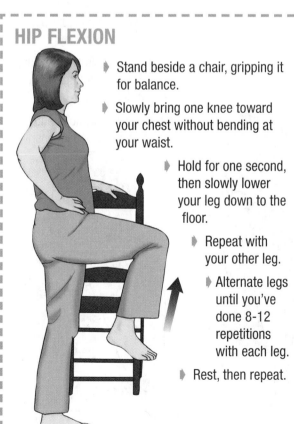

- ▸ Stand beside a chair, gripping it for balance.
- ▸ Slowly bring one knee toward your chest without bending at your waist.
  - ▸ Hold for one second, then slowly lower your leg down to the floor.
    - ▸ Repeat with your other leg.
    - ▸ Alternate legs until you've done 8-12 repetitions with each leg.
  - ▸ Rest, then repeat.

SIT TO STAND

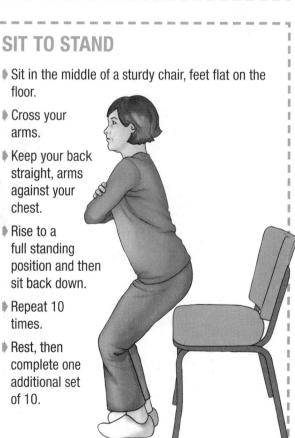

- ▸ Sit in the middle of a sturdy chair, feet flat on the floor.
- ▸ Cross your arms.
- ▸ Keep your back straight, arms against your chest.
- ▸ Rise to a full standing position and then sit back down.
- ▸ Repeat 10 times.
- ▸ Rest, then complete one additional set of 10.

SHOULDERS
Easy exercises help with shoulder pain

Nearly six million people a year see a doctor for some kind of shoulder problem. Three of the troublemakers—tendinitis, bursitis, and arthritis—are likely to develop with age, use, and overuse. It may be too late to prevent these problems, but it's never too late to keep them from getting worse and to ease the pain. These exercises can help stretch and strengthen your shoulders.

DUMBBELL OVERHEAD PRESS

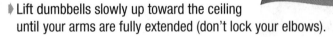

- ▶ Start with dumbbells you can comfortably lift for 8-12 repetitions.
- ▶ Hold one dumbbell in each hand at shoulder level, with elbows pointing down.
- ▶ Lift dumbbells slowly up toward the ceiling until your arms are fully extended (don't lock your elbows).
- ▶ Hold for 2 seconds, then lower slowly to the starting position.
- ▶ Repeat 8-12 times.

OVERHEAD REACH

- ▶ Standing, with your arms down, interlock your fingers in front of your lower abdomen.
- ▶ Lift your hands over your head and rotate your wrists so your palms are facing the sky.
- ▶ Extend your arms as far upward as possible and hold for 10 seconds, then return to the starting position.
- ▶ You should feel a stretch in the upper part of your back and in your shoulders.
- ▶ Repeat 2-3 times.

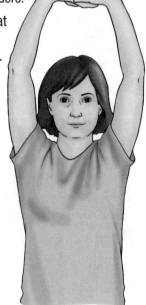

SHOULDER ROLL

- ▶ Standing position, arms down and at sides.
- ▶ Gently roll your shoulders back and down, trying to make your shoulder blades touch with each roll.
- ▶ 5-10 rotations, 2-3 sets.

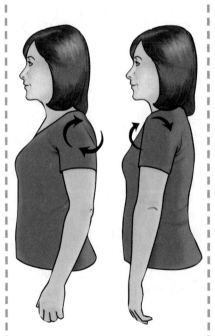

ELBOW PULLS

- ▶ Standing or sitting, place your left hand on your right shoulder.
- ▶ Grasp your left arm just above the elbow and pull your upper arm toward your body.
- ▶ Hold for 5 seconds, and then return to the starting position; repeat 8-12 times.
- ▶ Change arm positions and complete 8-12 repetitions.

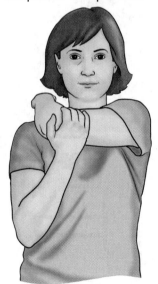

SHOULDER SQUEEZE

- Stand with elbows bent at your sides.
- Push your elbows back and squeeze your shoulder blades together.
- Hold for 10 seconds and then return to the starting position.
- Repeat 2-3 times.

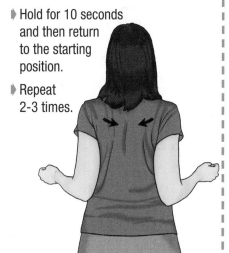

SHOULDER STRETCH

- Stand in front of an open doorway with your feet staggered.
- Raise your upper arms so that they are parallel to the floor.
- Place your palms against the frame of the door.
- Lean forward and hold the position for 10 seconds, and then return to the starting position.
- Repeat 2-3 times.

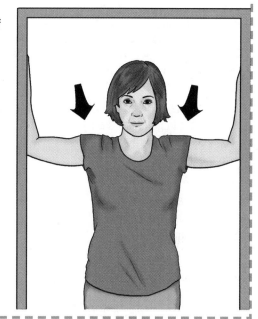

DUMBBELL KNEELING OVERHEAD PRESS

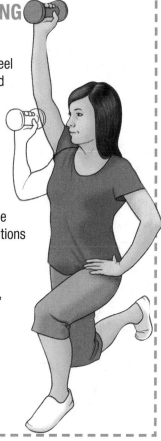

- Bend your left knee and kneel on your right knee, left hand on hip.
- Hold a 1-2 pound dumbbell in your right hand at shoulder height.
- Raise the dumbbell by straightening (but not locking) your arm toward the ceiling. Switch leg/arm positions and repeat on the other side.
- Work up to 8-10 repetitions, 2-3 sets for each arm.

Variation for beginners and older adults: Start with 4-5 repetitions, 1-2 sets.

DUMBBELL SHOULDER SHRUGS

- Stand with your feet a comfortable distance apart. Grasp a dumbbell in each hand, with your arms down and palms in toward your sides.
- Shrug your shoulders up and as high as possible.
- Hold for 1 second.
- Slowly return to the starting position and repeat.
- Perform 8 lifts at first (if you can, without pain) and gradually increase the number of repetitions to 12.

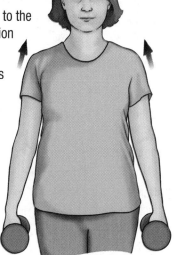

FINGERS & ANKLES

Easy exercises to ease finger and ankle stiffness

These range-of-motion exercises will ease stiffness and increase flexibility. If you suffer from finger or ankle arthritis, these exercises should be done every day.

FINGER EXTENSION

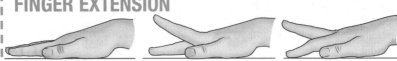

▶ Place your palm flat on the table. Then raise and lower each finger, one by one. Repeat 10 times.

ANKLE INVERSION

▶ Secure one end of a resistance band to a table leg or sturdy object, and hook the other end to the inside of your forefoot.

▶ Keep the heel still and move your forefoot inward, pulling against the band.

▶ Return to the starting position to complete 1 repetition.

▶ Complete 5-10 reps.

▶ After finishing your reps, switch feet and repeat.

THUMB OPPOSITION

▶ Begin by making an "O" by touching your thumb to each fingertip, one at a time. Do this 10 times with each finger.

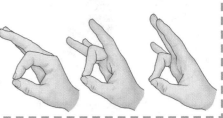

TENDON GLIDE

▶ Start with fingers together and your hand pointing straight up.

▶ Bend your fingers at the knuckles, pointing them forward and keeping them straight while your thumb still points upward. Hold for 5 seconds.

▶ Next, bend your thumb across your palm and bend your fingers at their midpoint, making a claw. Hold for 5 seconds.

▶ Finally, bend all your finger joints, drawing them into a full fist. Repeat this series 10 times with each hand.

ANKLE EVERSION

▶ Hook the band on the outside of your forefoot, and then move your foot to the outside against the band.

▶ Return to the starting position to complete 1 repetition.

▶ Complete 5-10 reps.

▶ After finishing your reps, switch feet and repeat.

ANKLE FLEX/EXTEND

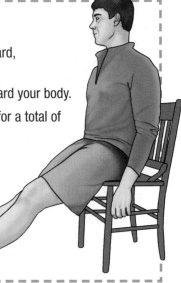

▶ In a sitting position, stretch your legs forward, heels on the floor.

▶ Flex your ankles, toes pointing up and toward your body.

▶ Hold for 10-30 seconds, relax, and repeat for a total of 2-3 repetitions, 1 set.

▶ Now flex your ankles, toes pointing down and away from your body.

▶ Hold for 10-30 seconds, relax, and repeat for a total of 2-3 repetitions, 1 set.

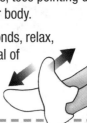

analgesic: a class of drugs that includes most painkillers

anesthesia: medication that causes partial or complete loss of sensation, and sometimes loss of consciousness

anesthetic: a medicine that temporarily blocks pain

anticonvulsant: a drug used to prevent seizures that also can treat pain

antidepressant: any type of medicine used to treat depression; some antidepressants are used to treat pain syndromes

autonomic nervous system: the part of the nervous system that regulates involuntary body functions (such as the heart, circulation, and body temperature)

bioelectric treatment: a procedure in which a precise dose of bioelectric current is administered through electrodes placed on the skin to cause a biological change and interrupt pain signals

biomarker: a characteristic that is measured and evaluated as an indicator of normal or disease process

capsaicin: a chemical found in chili peppers that is the primary ingredient in certain pain-relieving creams

central nervous system: the part of the nervous system made up of the brain and spinal cord

cognitive behavioral therapy: a method of therapy that attempts to correct ingrained patterns of negative behaviors and thoughts

corticosteroid (steroid): medication used to treat inflammation

cortisol: a hormone produced by the adrenal glands that decreases inflammation

COX-2 inhibitor: a nonsteroidal anti-inflammatory drug (NSAID) that is used to treat pain and reduce inflammation

discography: a procedure to determine whether an abnormal spinal disc is causing pain

drug pump: a device placed under the skin to deliver extremely small doses of medication, usually to the space around the spinal cord that contains fluid

endorphins: naturally occurring molecules that attach to receptors in the brain and spinal cord to stop pain messages

epidural: a procedure used to provide anesthesia during childbirth and some types of surgery

facet joint: a joint between two adjacent vertebrae

immune system: the system responsible for protecting the body from disease

inflammation: the response of body tissues to injury or irritation

intractable pain: pain that does not respond to treatment

intrathecal: fluid-containing space around the spinal cord

local anesthetic: a medication that blocks electrical signals and eliminates pain in a specific part of the body

myofascial pain: pain in the muscles and adjacent fibrous tissues

narcotics (opioids): drugs that relieve pain by preventing transmission of pain messages to the brain

nerve block: the use of drugs, chemical agents, or a surgical procedure to interrupt the transmission of pain messages

neuralgia: pain that extends along nerve pathways

neurolytic: a substance or procedure that destroys nerve tissue

neuropathic pain: pain caused by injury to or inflammation of the nerves

neurostimulation: electrical pulses delivered by an implanted device to stimulate the spinal cord

neurotransmitters: substances in the brain that carry signals between nerve cells

nociceptive (somatic) pain: pain caused by tissue damage in which chemicals are released and perceived by the brain as pain

nociceptor: a specialized nerve ending that senses unpleasant sensations

non-neuropathic pain: pain that does not involve nerve damage

nonsteroidal anti-inflammatory drug (NSAID): a drug used to reduce inflammation (aspirin, ibuprofen, and naproxen are examples)

opioids (narcotics): drugs that relieve pain by preventing transmission of pain messages to the brain (codeine, hydrocodone, and oxycodone are examples)

pain patch: a covering containing medication that is applied to the skin to relieve pain

pain receptor: a specialized nerve ending that identifies painful sensations and transmits them to a nerve

palliative care: treatment to relieve the pain, symptoms, and stress of serious illness, regardless of the diagnosis or prognosis

patient controlled analgesia (PCA): a system in which a person pushes a button and a machine delivers a dose of pain medicine into his or her bloodstream

peripheral nerve stimulation: a type of pain relief that uses electrical signals from an implanted device to stimulate nerves outside the spine

peripheral nervous system: the part of the nervous system that lies outside the brain and spinal cord

placebo: a harmless, inactive substance that has no direct effect on the cause of pain

sciatica: a condition caused by pressure on the sciatic nerve that causes pain in the buttocks, thighs, legs, ankles, and feet

serotonin: a chemical in the brain that helps to regulate mood

somatic (nociceptive) pain: pain caused by tissue damage in which chemicals are released and perceived by the brain as pain

spinal cord stimulation: electrical stimulation of nervous tissues in a specific portion of the spinal cord known as the dorsal column

spinal stenosis: narrowing of the canal surrounding the spinal cord

SSRIs (selective serotonin reuptake inhibitors): medications used to relieve depression that may also indirectly relieve pain

steroid: medication used to treat inflammation

subcutaneous: beneath the skin

sympathetic nervous system: one of two divisions of the autonomic nervous system that controls many of the involuntary activities of the glands, organs, and other parts of the body

syndrome: a group of symptoms that indicate a particular disorder

thalamus: the part of the brain that relays impulses from the nerves and enables people to feel pain

thermography: a measurement of heat produced by different parts of the body

topical drugs: medications that are applied to the skin

transdermal: a substance that enters the body through the skin

transcription therapy: treating conditions, including chronic pain, by introducing engineered genes into a patient's cells

tricyclic antidepressants: a group of drugs used to relieve symptoms of depression that may also relieve pain

trigger point: a specific spot that is painful to touch or pressure

X-STOP: a minimally invasive procedure in which an implant is used to maintain the space between the spinous processes to prevent pressure on the nerves while standing

APPENDIX III: RESOURCES

For more information on arthritis:

American Academy of Orthopaedic Surgeons
www.aaos.org
847-823-7186
9400 West Higgins Rd., Rosemont, IL 60018

American College of Rheumatology
www.rheumatology.org
Email: acr@rheumatology.org
404-633-3777
2200 Lake Blvd., NE, Atlanta, GA 30319

American Pain Society
www.americanpainsociety.org
Email: info@americanpainsociety.org
847-375-4715
8735 W. Higgins Rd., Suite 300, Chicago, IL 60631

The Arthritis Foundation
www.arthritis.org
Email: help@arthritis.org
404-872-7100
Mail: 1330 West Peachtree St., Ste.
100, Atlanta, GA 30309

**National Institute of Arthritis
and Musculoskeletal and Skin Diseases:**
Information Clearinghouse
www.niams.nih.gov
Email: niamsinfo@mail.nih.gov
877-226-4267
301-495-4484
1 AMS Circle, Bethesda, MD 20892-3675

National Institute on Aging Information Center
www.nia.nih.gov
Email: niaic@nia.nih.gov
800-222-2225
Building 31, Room 5C27
31 Center Drive, MSC 2292, Bethesda, MD 20892

FDA/Drug Information Pathfinder
www.fda.gov/cder/
Extensive list of links to all things related to medications, including over-the-counter, prescription, and experimental

Medline Plus/Arthritis
www.nlm.nih.gov/medlineplus/arthritis.html
A rich source of information on arthritis (and other diseases and conditions) from the National Library of Medicine. Lots of links to the latest news, medication lists, research studies, treatment options, and statistics.

American Society of Health-System Pharmacists
www.safemedication.com
301-657-3000
7272 Wisconsin Avenue, Bethesda MD 20814
Easy-to-read info on more than 800 prescribed medications and how to use them wisely.

The Cochrane Library
www.cochrane.org
The Cochrane Library is a collection of science-based reviews from the Cochrane Collaboration, an international nonprofit organization. Its authors analyze the results of rigorous clinical trials on a given topic and prepare summaries called systematic reviews. Abstracts of these reviews can be read on the Web without charge.

For more information on living with arthritis:

American Occupational Therapy Association, Inc.
www.aota.org
301-652-6611
4720 Montgomery Lane, Suite 20
Bethesda, MD 20814-3449

Aids for Arthritis, Inc.
www.aidsforarthritis.com
800-654-0707

Comfort House
www.comforthouse.com
800-359-7701

APPENDIX III: RESOURCES

For products to make living with arthritis easier:

Disability Travel and Recreation Resources
www.makoa.org/travel.htm
Large list of links to all things related
to traveling with disability

American Orthotic Prosthetic Association
www.aopanet.org
Email: info@AOPAnet.org
571-431-0876
Orthotic Patient Education
330 John Carlyle Street, Ste. 200, Alexandria, VA 22314

Access-Able Travel Source
www.access-able.com
Email: information@access-able.com
303-232-2979
PO Box 1796, Wheat Ridge, CO 80034
Database of information and resources
for travelers with special needs.

Food and Diet Advice
www.choosemyplate.gov
This website, put together by the U.S. Department
of Agriculture, explains the 2010 Dietary Guidelines
for Americans and gives interactive assistance in
helping you decide what and how much to eat.

For more information on complementary and alternative medicine:

American Academy of Medical Acupuncture
www.medicalacupuncture.org
310-364-0193
1970 E. Grand Ave., Suite 330, El Segundo, CA 90245

American Massage Therapy Association
www.amtamassage.org
Email: info@amtamassage.com
877-905-0577
500 Davis Street, Ste. 900, Evanston, IL 60201

National Center for Complementary and Integrative Health
www.nccih.nih.gov
Email: info@nccih.nih.gov
888-644-6226
9000 Rockville Pike, Bethesda, MD 20892

The American Yoga Association
www.americanyogaassociation.org/contents.html
Email: info@americanyogaassociation.org
P.O. Box 19986, Sarasota, FL 34276

REPORT: NIH Research Project Database
http://projectreporter.nih.gov/reporter.cfm
REPORT (Research Portfolio Online Reporting
Tools) is a searchable database of federally
funded biomedical research projects conducted at
universities, hospitals, and other research institutions.
Simply enter the name of an herb, supplement,
medication, or institution into the search form.

Natural Medicines Comprehensive Database
http://www.naturaldatabase.com/
This is a fee-based database used by physicians
and others to find information on the latest
clinical studies on natural medicines.

National Certification Commission
for Acupuncture and Oriental Medicine
www.nccaom.org
904-598-1005
76 S. Laura St., Suite 1290, Jacksonville, FL 32202

U.S. Food and Drug Administration (FDA)/MedWatch
www.fda.gov/medwatch/report/consumer/consumer.htm
888-463-6332
MedWatch is the FDA's safety information and adverse
event reporting program. Consumers or health care
providers may file a report on a serious problem that
they suspect is associated with a dietary supplement.

FDA Food Safety
http://www.fda.gov/Food/default.htm

Office of Dietary Supplements (ODS), NIH
http://ods.od.nih.gov
The ODS supports and disseminates research in
the area of dietary supplements. It produces the
International Bibliographic Information on Dietary
Supplements (IBIDS) database on the Web, which
contains citations to and abstracts of peer-reviewed
scientific literature on dietary supplements.